*"What is flirting?"*
*"Should people of different religions date each other?"*
*"How can I break up with my boyfriend and still be friends?"*
*"I've lost my virginity. Can God forgive me?"*

These questions, and others like them, are important to teenagers, who must make choices every day of their lives — choices that will affect the *rest* of their lives. In order to make these vital decisions, they need facts, background information, understanding, and motivation.

Barry Wood knows the questions teenagers ask. His answers are honest and open, based on biblical principles that have been tested and found to be valid.

This is a book that will give young people firm footing as they choose their paths through today's morass of morality.

BY Barry Wood

*Questions Non-Christians Ask*
*Questions New Christians Ask*
*Questions Teenagers Ask About Dating and Sex*

# Questions Teenagers Ask About Dating and Sex

Barry Wood

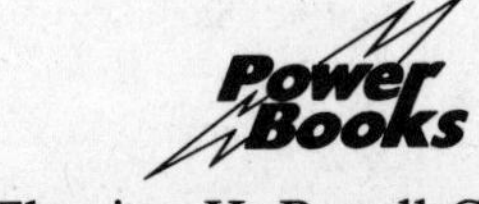


Fleming H. Revell Company
Old Tappan, New Jersey

Library of Congress Cataloging in Publication Data

Wood, Barry, date
Questions teenagers ask about dating and sex.

Summary: Addresses dating, marriage, sex, love, and other topics that concern teenage Christians.
1. Sex instruction for youth. 2. Dating (Social customs) [1. Conduct of life. 2. Sex instruction for youth] I. Title.
HQ35.W64 306.7 81-2704
ISBN 0-8007-5058-6 AACR2


Published by Fleming H. Revell Company

Printed in the United States of America

TO

the thousands of teenagers who have asked me *their* questions. Without them, this could not have been written. Many thanks for their courage to ask the "unaskable" questions.

# Contents

## SEX



## LOVE

# Preface

The Sexual Revolution of the last decade has now gone full circle. The sexual habits of the adult community have now reached into high school and junior-high school. The youth of this generation are moving into the 1980s sexually wise and morally confused. You'd think that after twenty years of sex education in the public schools, today's teenagers would be the most enlightened and responsible youth this nation has ever produced. Not so. The truth is, sex education is a failure in most instances. One million teenage girls get pregnant each year. That's a startling one out of every ten! Permissiveness is the hallmark of the teen culture. Johns Hopkins University spent eight years conducting a survey of teenagers' sexual habits. Professors Melvin Zelnik and John F. Kantner reveal that nearly 50 percent of America's young women between fifteen and nineteen years of age are no longer virgins. What is shocking about these statistics is that the percentage has doubled since 1971 when the survey began!

Sex education has not helped stem the tide of increased venereal disease. Teenagers account for 25 percent of all reported cases of gonorrhea each year. Even though most teenagers have been taught about birth control, 80 percent of all sexually active teenagers fail to use contraceptives! Something's wrong somewhere! Maybe the answer's found in the statement of a seventeen-year-old youth made to me recently: "My sex-education class has shown me the 'how' of sex, but it has not given me the 'why' of sex." This is tragically true. Teaching young people about sex without teaching them about moral values should be considered a crime! Dr. Frank Furshenberg, Jr., a sociologist from the University of Pennsylvania, remarked in a *Newsweek* article, "It's safe to teach the mechanics of reproduction, but threatening to talk about values and responsibilities." (Read this revealing September 1, 1980, article "Teenage Sex: The New Morality Hits Home.") Indeed, in many public-school systems teachers are forbidden to teach sexual values and morals.

Because of these rather shocking facts, we have felt the need for a book such as this. As we travel America, speaking in school assemblies and teaching dating and sex seminars, we find that teenagers are asking questions as to the *why* of sex. They are in desperate need of some guidelines and a moral structure to live by.

The questions in this book go beyond the classic big four: *homosexuality, abortion, oral sex,* and *masturbation.* These questions are always asked everywhere I go. However, there are other questions that teenagers everywhere ask. Some of them sound juvenile to an adult mind, but they are *real* questions and they demand real answers. We hope our answers go beyond Dear Abby! The advice we give will be based on biblical insights, because today's youth very much need a word from God on the subjects of dating, love, and sex. Make no mistake about it, God does have some very practical things to say about sex. After all, He is *the* authority on the subject—He invented it! Right?

So, here are our answers to the questions teenagers have asked in over one hundred seminars across the land. May the Lord bless the application of these answers to some teenagers' lives in order that dating and sex become a blessing and not a curse.

BARRY WOOD

# DATING

*It matters not that the whole world rejects me if the inner circle of my brothers and sisters in Christ accept me and give me support to carry through.*

*Martin Luther King, Jr.*

# 1 Can You Define Dating for Me?

**MY PARENTS DO NOT THINK I AM OLD ENOUGH TO DATE. I TELL THEM THAT I'M NOT READY TO "DATE" BUT I DO LIKE TO BE WITH GUYS, BUT OUR TIME TOGETHER ISN'T A "DATE." HOW DO YOU DEFINE DATING, AND IS THERE SUCH A THING AS JUST BEING FRIENDS?**

The young lady who wrote this letter to me has my total sympathy. Yes, you can "just be friends" and not all boy-girl relationships have to be dating relationships. Dating is not the way to *make* friends. Christians are not candidates for dating clubs, where you send in your stats for a computer readout and they match you up with your clone!

Yet, some parents and well-meaning friends get pushy about this. Kids get pushed into "dating" by the various Cupids of our society who love to play matchmaker.

### *Dating by Barry*

Christian young people and their parents need to think through this dating business, because if you don't, the world and its philosophy will do the thinking for you. Today's youth culture desperately needs guidance in its dating habits. Too many guys and gals have the mistaken concept that dating is where you practice your sex technique. You know—it's like the preseason where you practice for the "league" play. Dating is where you learn to be a lover, and really "put the moves" on each other. Well, that may be the way it's done by the masses, but that's not God's way. God's way of dating is infinitely superior. He only deals in the best. He wants His children to have super sex and dynamic dating. As the saying goes, "God don't sponsor no flops!" He doesn't want your dating to be a flop. Therefore, we must look at dating differently. We've taught Christian dating standards to thousands of young people, and these standards have proved to be very practical.

### *A Special Friendship*

What is dating? I define dating as "a special kind of friendship between two people of the opposite sex that may lead to courtship, love, and marriage." Notice, dating is a friendship, a *special kind* of friendship. Courtship—all that romantic stuff—should come *after* a very special friendship has developed. Too often couples become lovers before becoming friends. It shouldn't be that way. Strangers and lovers make odd couples. What is needed is the concept that two people of the opposite sex can have a nonphysical, nonromantic friendship which is growing in spiritual oneness. For my part, dating is to be reserved for those special friendships. You should not date anyone who isn't *already* a close or intimate friend.

### *Close Friends Have Freedom*

What are the characteristics of a close friendship? I define a close friendship as one in which there is freedom to discuss vital issues without fear of rejection; such vital issues include spiritual goals like salvation and God's will. There is freedom also to work on and discuss spiritual growth; that is, prayer, the Bible, and mutual efforts to help each other grow spiritually. Often a young woman, asking me to perform a wedding ceremony, admits she doesn't even know if her fiancé is a Believer! What shocks me more is that she thinks she loves him! How can she love him? She hardly *knows* him. That's right, you can't really know a person without a close friendship that allows for freedom to discuss the real issues in life. Those issues are: *Who is God? Who am I? Why am I here? What is God's plan for my life?* Until two people have waded through the muddy waters of these issues together, they haven't really touched each other's souls. Dating (physical romantic relationships) only hinders this kind of communication if it precedes it.

***Intimate Friends Are Committed***

Intimate friends are even closer. They have become so close that they are committed to each other's growth. Intimate friends are walking together toward Christlikeness. Character development is the natural result of their time together.

If friends of the opposite sex would develop this kind of growing friendship, the dating would take care of itself. You see, dating grows out of the friendship. When a friendship starts to become a courtship, dating has begun. That's the way it should be. That's the best way; it's God's way. Did you know the Bible does not say one single word about dating? Makes you wonder why. Perhaps because it is not in His plan. He does affirm and encourage friendship. He does admonish sexual purity and discourage impurity among single people. It leads me to believe that God sees dating as sort of preengagement reserved for very special friendships. What do you think?

# 2 Does God Really Have Just One Special Person Picked Out for Me?

Now here's a question we've all thought about somewhere in our romantic youth: "Is there a special person, my Prince Charming or Princess Grace, just waiting for me?" I know I spent some hours daydreaming about "that" girl as a young teenager. Who hasn't? Yet, even more real is the question of God's concern for our sexual-social needs. Is His will for His children's lives so specific that He even plays matchmaker for us? Surely God has more important things to do! or does He?

It is Jesus who teaches us about His Father's concern for us. He said, "Do not be anxious then, saying, 'What shall we eat?' or 'What shall we drink?' or 'With what shall we clothe ourselves?' . . . for your heavenly Father knows that you need all these things" (Matthew 6:31,32). So you see, God is concerned about our basic needs—food, clothes, the daily things. It follows then that He desires to provide for our spiritual needs—those needs that only a life companion can meet. He did so for Adam in the Garden of Eden. God brought Eve into Adam's life, in order that Adam might be fulfilled. I believe God will do the same for each of us who trust Him for it.

However, does that mean that God has one specific person picked out for each of us? Not necessarily. First of all, it is not

God's plan that every one of us marry. There is a plan for singleness in His Kingdom. One girl heard me say that and exclaimed, "Dear God, I hope it's not me!" Rest assured that if it is His plan for you, you will be given grace for that kind of life. He did so for the apostle Paul. (*See* 1 Corinthians 7:7,8.) Some Christians have remained single in order to have freedom for ministry. Tradition has indicated this was God's plan for the apostle Paul.

Yet, if God does intend marriage for you, He no doubt desires to bring that right person into your life. Certainly He knows whom you need. However, to say that there is only *one* specific person just may not be accurate. What if you marry and your husband dies, can God bring another Prince Charming into your life? What do we call him—Prince Charming II?

I know a wonderful Christian man who is seventy-nine years old at this writing. He's outlived two wives and is considering his third! He'd tell you each of his gals was God's special one for *that time* in his life. So you see, if you live long enough, God might give you half a dozen—one at a time!

Well, that's silly, but be sure to get my point. Yes, God's will for us does include the details of whom we date, fall in love with, and perhaps marry. His love is that specific. The question then arises, "How do I know when I've found the right one?" That's coming up next—and it's very exciting!

# 3 How Can I Know for Sure I've Found the Right Person?

It was just about twenty-four hours before the wedding. The phone rang at my home about 8:00 P.M. When I answered, I heard a crying female voice on the line. It was Jill, the bride-to-be for tomorrow's wedding. She was very frightened. When finally I calmed her down enough to talk coherently, she told me the source of her distress. Jill said, "How do I know for sure he's the right one for me? I think I love him, but I have these terrible doubts!" Such doubts can be very real. Jill's were so real she cancelled the wedding at great cost and embarrassment to her and the others involved.

Jill never did marry that guy. Maybe you shouldn't either—I mean *your* guy or girl. Maybe he or she's not the one for you. Perhaps God has someone else in mind for you. How can you know for sure? Believe me, there's no simple answer to that question. Far too many couples with stars in their eyes have marched down the aisle, cut the cake, and really believed it was "till death do us part." Later he or she discovered that the spouse turned out to be someone very different from what he/she had thought. Mr. or Mrs. "Right" turned out to be Mr. or Mrs. "Wrong."

In answer to this question, I'm going to avoid the kindred question, "How can I know when I'm in love?" because that area is discussed elsewhere in this book. For now, let's think about how to find the right person for you. I assume we mean the right person for "life." You know: for love, marriage, and family; that's what is usually meant.

To begin with, let me ask you a fundamental question. By the *right* person, do you mean the *best* person? It seems that too often where dating is concerned, we settle for less than the best. God only deals in the best. He knows nothing of what's average, popular, cute, handsome, or pretty. He *wants* you to have the best. So the *right* girl, or the *right* guy, from God's perspective, means that person who is the best for you. Are you willing to wait for the best? Do you really want God's very best for dates, and later—marriage? Because if you're not committed to the best, Satan will see to it that you settle for less.

A few years ago a lovely young lady came to my office for counselling. She was about twenty-three years old, a high-school English teacher, and very single, very lonely. No sooner had she sat down to talk, than the tears began to roll down her cheeks. I asked her to share with me what was bothering her. Her reply really touched my heart, yet I had to restrain myself to keep from laughing. Through her tears she said, with much emphasis, "I need a man! I'm tired of being alone. I haven't had a real date in months, and don't want to stay single the rest of my life." There she was—a thoroughly frustrated single woman! Have you ever felt like that? Just about everybody has! What advice would you give her? Because you see, this young lady is a very mature Christian. She taught a Sunday-school class of college women; she is a witness for Christ. Yet, even spiritual people have sexual/social needs. She needed a companion!

### *Only the Best*

My counsel to her just may help you. I asked her a few questions, such as, "Well, Susan, what kind of man are you looking for? If God isn't meeting your needs [in dating], then there's got to be a good reason for it." Susan asked, "What do you mean, what kind of guy am I looking for? Do you mean, like tall, dark and handsome?" "No, no," I replied. "I mean what type of person would you fall in love with? What spiritual characteristics would you require of your man?" I then got out a pencil and note pad and asked her to describe her future lover. Thoughtfully, Susan began to name those characteristics, as I wrote them down—a mature Christian, a spiritual leader who loves God and His Word, who is kind, thoughtful, and on and on she went. I had to tell her to slow down, so I could list them! It soon became very apparent to me that she had really given much thought to this. She had her man all picked out—and what a man he was. He was a combination of Robert Redford, John Travolta, Francis of Assisi, and the apostle Paul! She wanted only the best, and that's good! I wish more single people did want only the best.

### *Getting the Best*

Breathless, I said to her, "Well, now, it seems to me that you've given God quite an order to fill. No wonder you're still single; you've eliminated about ninety-five percent of the male species! It will take God more time to find a guy to satisfy you, young lady!" I was teasing, of course, but I was also excited for her. Now all that remained was for her to figure out how to get God to bring her Prince Charming a-callin.'

At this point, I asked Susan a direct question. "If God were to bring this fine young man into your life right now, would you be good for him? Would you be a blessing to him, or would you be a mismatch?" Susan looked at me rather puzzled and replied, "I don't know. I never thought about it before." "Well, think about it," I said. She did, then said softly, "No, I'm probably not ready for a man like that." Reluctantly I told her, "Susan, there is your answer. God has not provided a man for you for two reasons. First, you've set your goals very high and that's terrific; but God knows you're not ready. When He sees you are truly worthy of such a man, He'll bring him into your life." And, my dear reader, this is so true. It is one of God's principles of life that in order to get the best you must become the best. God will not "unequally yoke" two people together (2 Corinthians 6:14 KJV). He's a perfect matchmaker. Gini Andrews, in her great little book for girls, says, "Let's be brutally honest: if you do run across this dreamboat of yours, what makes you so sure he'll fall for you?" That's a good question. (Read Gini Andrews's *Your Half of the Apple,* pages 41–50, for a good discussion of the virtuous woman in Proverbs 31.)

### *Finding God's Best*

Susan is a married woman today, and she got the guy of her dreams. She met him about a year or so later. She did so by following the advice I'm about to give you. I'll tell you what I told her about finding that "right" person.

### *Believe God Will Provide for You*

First, you don't have to shop around and date three different people each week. Save your time and money for other things. God said in Romans 8:32 that He would provide for your needs. Trust Him to do it. Don't stick your nose in His business. Pray about it continually, and really believe God will provide.

### *Determine to Settle for Nothing Less Than the Best*

Second, like Susan, set your sights high. You want Mr. (Miss) Terrific. Beware of Satan's substitutes. He'll sure tempt you to settle for less.

### *Seek to Become the Best Yourself*

Rather than flirting, dating, and being sexually aggressive by "shopping around," spend quality time becoming a quality person. To get a godly mate, become godly yourself. That's what Susan did. She redoubled her efforts to become a better woman, to make herself more attractive (inside) to that man God was preparing for her.

***Know That When the Timing Is Right, God Will Provide***

When God sees that each of you is ready for a mature courtship, He will initiate circumstances to bring you together. He can and will do it. You may be a little suspicious of my theology about now. I can hear you saying, "Hey, how do I know you're telling me the truth?" I doubt that you've ever thought about it, but this advice I've given you comes right out of the Garden of Eden—that's how old it is. Think about God's provision for His son Adam's need.

God the Father knew that Adam needed a companion long before Adam did. I doubt Adam knew *what* he needed! He'd never seen a woman or had any idea what sex was all about. He didn't know what or who he needed to be fulfilled, but His Heavenly Father knew! You and I are like that—we think we know who we need—"I need *her*" or "I need *him,*" but so often we are wrong.

Then, notice that God met Adam's need by creating Eve. She was perfect woman for perfect man. I'm certain that Adam didn't complain! She was all he could have hoped for and more. God will provide for you as He did for Adam. However, there is a condition: You and I have to trust Him to do it. Adam allowed God to "cause a deep sleep" to come over him. Trusting in God, Adam permitted God to create Eve out of his side (a rib, I believe it was). So, you see, what God did then He continues to do for children who trust Him. "For He performs what is appointed for me, And many such decrees are with Him" (Job 23:14).

# 4 Is It Okay for People of Two Different Religions to Date? Marry?

A question like this is most often asked *after* the fact. When you're already dating someone of a "different religion," you become acutely aware of the very real differences between you.

I met a college girl a few years ago who was dating a very wealthy, tall, dark, and handsome Arab guy. It didn't take too many dates for her to discover that his approach to dating (women) was not what she was accustomed to. He wanted to make her a part of his harem! His concept of womanhood was influenced by his Islamic religion. Needless to say, it didn't work out for this Christian girl and her sheik. Religious differences can become *the* difference in a relationship.

***Religions and Denominations***

Can a couple have a good dating relationship—and even a marriage—if their religions are different? Perhaps, but first we need to be more specific about what you mean by "religion." There is a very clear distinction between Christian denominations and "other" religions. For example, a Protestant and a Catholic do not belong to two different religions. Neither do Baptists and Lutherans worship two different Gods. Within the

Christian family there are many groups of believers we call denominations. (The term *denomination* is normally applied to groups within the Protestant and evangelical Christian families.) These denominations share a common body of agreed-upon doctrine based upon the Bible. They agree as to who Jesus is, why He came into the world, what He did for us on the Cross, and how, through faith in Him, we can have the forgiveness of sins and peace with God. This common thread of belief makes all those who put their faith in Christ brothers and sisters, regardless of which Christian church groups they belong to. However, there can be some very real problems when Christians of differing cultures marry—more about that later.

However, other so-called religions can be described as those non-Christian religions that seek to find relationship with God *without* belief in God's Son, Jesus Christ. Some of these faiths dress in the garb of Christian appearance but are not Christian at all.

### *The Christian and Cults*

Without being too technical, we do need to explain the difference between a Christian denomination and a Christian cult. A young person who is a Christian may understand that a Moslem, Buddhist, or Hindu does not believe about God and Christ the way he does; but may not comprehend that Mormons, Jehovah's Witnesses, Christian Scientists, and others also do *not* believe about God and Christ the way he does. Mistakenly, he may assume that these groups are also Christian and part of the mainline Christian faith.

Not too long ago, a college-age young man told me he was in love with a Mormon girl. He also told me that he was a member of an Independent Bible Church and that there was very little difference between what his church teaches and what his girl believes (as a Mormon)! Now that's incredibly naive! That guy either knows very little about what he believes or very little about what his Mormon girl friend believes—or both! Either way, their beliefs are *not* compatible—not at all.

### *Cults Are Not Christian*

Understand this: A "cult" is not Christian even though they talk the language. You may be asking, "What is a cult?" It may be an oversimplified answer, but a cult is any organized group that claims to be Christian, but its teachings deny crucial truth about who Jesus is and why He came. They usually deny Christ's deity as God. God's Word warns us to beware of those who deny Jesus His place as God's Son, our Savior.

> Beloved, do not believe every spirit, but test the spirits to see whether they are from God; because many false prophets have gone out into the world. By this you know the Spirit of God: every spirit that confesses that Jesus Christ has come in the flesh is from God; and every spirit that does not confess Jesus is not from God; and this is the spirit of the antichrist.
>
> 1 John 4:1–3

This warning must be heeded by those in a dating relationship, because in an affair of the heart, the heart rules the head! Your head may tell you, "My boyfriend isn't a Christian, and I shouldn't continue this courtship because it doesn't please the Lord, and it can never work." However, the heart doesn't react that way. The heart says, "My boyfriend isn't a Christian, but our love will overcome all barriers. We'll work it out." Too many times couples lead with their hearts, only to have their hearts broken later on. *Religious beliefs are important.*

### *Plan Ahead*

What I suggest is simply this. Plan ahead. Know what you believe. Take time to discover God in His Word for yourself. Stick your own individual nose into your own individual Bible! Then, when you have formed some convictions, promise yourself and

God that you will seek to live by those convictions. Because you are a Christian, Jesus Christ and His Will should come first in your date life. Give your future dating relationships to Him. Ask His guidance daily.

### *Before It Goes Too Far*

Then, whenever you start dating someone regularly, begin to discuss spiritual things together. Find out where he or she is "coming from." This should be a normal part of getting to know each other. Find out what each of you believes *before* a romance starts.

A college girl came to my office a few years ago, wanting me to preside over her wedding. She was a senior in college, planning marriage right after graduation. Her boyfriend was also a senior. I asked her if she was a Christian. Replying excitedly, she said, "Oh, yes, I come to hear you preach every Sunday!" I then asked her about her fiancé's relationship to Christ. She very defensively said, "Oh, we never discuss religion. My boyfriend says there are two things a man doesn't want a woman to talk about—religion and politics!" Well, what do you think about that? You can imagine *my* reaction. Wow! I nearly exploded! This poor girl was willing to marry a guy who refused to talk to her about the *real* issues of life. The truth was—they hardly knew one another. Their relationship was shallow and based mostly on physical attraction. It was too late for that couple.

### *The Common Denominator*

After spending time together in a noncourtship kind of friendship, you may discover that the two of you have much in common in your beliefs. Even though you don't go to the same kind of church, you feel you both are born-again Christians. This is the most important issue between you. Since both of you really love Jesus, then you can openly discuss your faith. Seek to discover if the differences between your beliefs are major or minor.

Would they affect your future relationship should you fall in love? If the differences are very real, should you stop dating because of them? Sometimes the answer is an obvious *yes.*

### *A Family Affair*

Remember, serious dating and then marriage is a family affair. You don't just marry a person—you marry his whole tribe. You marry his "roots." Suppose you are a Baptist and your family is deeply committed to their Baptist faith. Suppose your boyfriend (girl friend) is a Catholic and his/her family are deeply devoted to their Catholic faith. Do you and your lover have problems? You bet your life you do!

Only three weeks ago I found this very problem as a counselor. A young married couple was facing a crisis. She is Baptist; he is Catholic. His brother is a priest, and his family has been Catholic for generations. He wants her to have a child; she wants one also but refuses to have one because she doesn't want her baby to be baptized into the Catholic church. His parents insist the child be baptized. The young husband resents his wife's taking the Pill for birth control; he doesn't believe in it; she does. They never discussed these future problems when they were dating. Her father is a Baptist preacher and has had a very difficult time accepting the marriage. The two families are at war over this couple. When they finally came to me for counselling, they were near divorce, which neither of them really wanted or believed in. What would you tell them to do? It's a tough situation that may or may not work out but it could have been prevented. *Listen to me*—foresight is better than hindsight. An ounce of prevention is worth a pound of cure (to quote my grandmother).

### *The Long and the Short*

My best advice to teens is to take the long look—not just the short look—when dating. Realize you never know when or with whom you'll fall in love. Make up your mind *beforehand* what kind of person you are looking for. Plan for the future. When you date, make Christ a part of your date life from the beginning, and things will turn out for the best.

*I'm in with the "IN" crowd*
*I go where the "IN" crowd goes,*

*We've got our way of walkin'*
*We've got our way of talkin'*

*Spendin' cash*
*and talkin' trash!*

# 5 How Can I Keep From Following the Crowd in My Date Life?

**MANY OF MY GIRL FRIENDS GET MORE DATES THAN I DO BECAUSE THEY "FOOL AROUND" A LOT WITH THE GUYS. I'M AGAINST PETTING AND OTHER PHYSICAL INVOLVEMENT, BUT I DO WANT TO GO OUT WITH NICE GUYS. HOW CAN I KEEP FROM FOLLOWING THE CROWD IN MY DATE LIFE?**

Peer pressure. That's what it's called. (Peer pressure—your "peers" are those people in your life who are your equals, your companions. Peer pressure is what we call "following the crowd." *See also* Glossary.) Everyone has to deal with it, especially single young people. The temptation to "follow the crowd" in your dating habits is a very real temptation. As one young girl said, "You either go along or you don't go at all!"

Christian young people must face the pressure of group behavior. "Everybody's doing it" is the theme song of many teenagers. Moral decisions are then made on the basis of what's *in* rather than what is eternally right or wrong. In some high schools more girls are non-virgins than virgins. The sixteen-year-old virgin is pressured to have sex just to prove herself a woman. One girl told me she had sex "just to get it over with." Young men face an even greater pressure to score with numerous girls to prove their prowess.

Much of this peer pressure is Satan-inspired to trap you. Satan can lead you astray through dating and sex. He likes you to date the wrong person and to determine your sexual behavior by your culture, rather than by Christ's teachings. He uses peer pressure to determine whom you date, where you go on a date, and how you will behave on a date. The Bible warns us to beware of peer pressure when it says, "Don't let the world around you squeeze you into its own mould . . ." (Romans 12:2 PHILLIPS). How can a Christian young person resist this squeeze play? It is not easy to stand alone in your date life. Standing alone just may mean staying alone or staying at home!

### *What Is Popularity?*

Often we do things sexually that we know are wrong just because we think we're expected to. A girl wants to be popular with the boys. A guy wants the ladies to like him. However, we just may be confused about what popularity *really* is. I've known teenagers who thought "getting attention" and being popular were synonymous. Not so! A girl can play it loose sexually with every boy she dates, and you can bet she'll get lots of attention! Boys will date her for what she does to them and with them. They will not date her for what she is. *Popularity* is the result of what you are; *attention* is the result of what you do. You can cuss and get attention. You can get drunk and get attention. You can do crazy things to make people laugh and get attention. However, these things do not mean you are popular.

### *Steps to Popularity*

I like to help young people understand how to become popular with their peers. This is very important because those who are popular can be leaders and pacesetters with their friends. He who is popular can turn peer pressure into peer power. He who has peer power puts peer pressure on others. That's the only way to fly! All right, what are the steps to popularity?

*Achievement.* The first step to popularity is *achievement.* As a young person, find something worth doing and do it well. Excel at something worthwhile, such as sports, school, music, and so on. Discipline yourself until you are one of the best at what you do. Others will begin to notice you for your accomplishment.

Recently I attended a marathon race with a friend of mine who is a runner (I'm a jogger; there is a *big* difference). At this race I met Sean Hartley. Sean is an 11-year-old marathon runner. He holds the world records in the 9, 10, and 11-year-old divisions of the 26-mile, 385-yard marathon run. After the race, when about 25 young girls were circled around young Sean, I asked his father, "What makes Sean work so hard at his running?" Mr. Hartley replied, pointing at the circle of girls and his smiling son, "Good point. Popularity is the result of achievement."

*Respect.* The second step in being popular is *respect.* Because of what you and I achieve, others will respect us. It is more important that your friends *respect* you than it is that they *like* you. Jesus Himself was not liked or loved by all men. However, all men respected Him. Even His enemies respected Him. That should be our goal. Girls, in your dating, do the boys you date respect you? Do they really? Do you demand that respect? The same questions apply to you young men. Respect from others is often the result of your achievements or character commitments. Because of what you accomplish, you are respected; then as a result of this respect, you are popular. You then have peer power over your friends.

### *Standing Alone*

Don't misunderstand me. It can cost you points with the crowd if you don't go along. Following Jesus definitely has its drawbacks for the committed disciple. Jesus predicted for us, "In the world you will have tribulation" (*see* John 16:33). Therefore, you may just as well make up your mind to go it alone at times.

Sexual behavior for the Christian probably won't be what's in among teens in your school. It will help you cope with the problem if you resolve early in your teen years to stand alone, if need be, rather than compromise your morals.

### *The Road to Peer Power*

Indeed, standing alone just may be the only way to become a leader. When a person stands alone for his or her convictions, that person is shouting to the world that there are values worth standing for. Those who follow the crowd take the low road and influence very few. Those who stand alone are respected and often become attractive to others. Standing alone develops leadership and character in one's self. So you see, *not* following the crowd *can* have its benefits. Popularity, respect, leadership, can be your reward. Why not be the one who marches to a different drummer in your sex life?

### *A Threefold Result*

Finally, then, here is a threefold result of resisting peer pressure in your date life. *First,* your friends will realize whose side you are on. They will know you belong to Christ, not the crowd. *Second,* you are learning to be your own self. *Third,* God sees He can trust you and therefore will bless and use you. That's really neat! In your date life you can be used of God to strengthen many others by refusing to lower your standards.

Suggested Reading

Hartley, Fred. *Dare to Be Different: Dealing With Peer Pressure.* Old Tappan, NJ: Power Books (Revell), 1980.

# 6 Does Age Make Any Difference in Dating?

**MY BOYFRIEND IS SEVERAL YEARS OLDER THAN I AM, AND MY PARENTS DON'T WANT ME TO DATE HIM. DOES AGE MAKE ANY DIFFERENCE IN DATING?**

I proposed marriage to my first girl friend. I was five years old and she was four. She turned me down. I asked her why. She told me that they only marry relatives in her family. I was confused and asked her to explain. She did. In her four-year-old wisdom she said, "Well, my mommy married my daddy, my grandma married my grandpa, and my aunts all married my uncles!" Smart girl! Well, does age have something to do with dating and marriage?

The girl who wrote this question didn't tell me what her own age is, or the age of her boyfriend. That *does* make a difference, especially if she is only four! Surely there is an age that is too young to begin to date, and surely there is an age difference that is too great to be healthy and good.

### *When Are You Old Enough to Date?*

To begin with, there is a minimum age for dating. In our seminars we ask teenagers to list the age they think is acceptable to begin dating. It's very revealing that all the thirteen-year-olds think they are old enough, and all the fourteen-year-olds think they are too. My guess is that if we let twelve-year-olds attend the dating seminar they too would think they are ready! Often young teens lack objectivity. Here are some suggestions to determine when is an acceptable age to begin dating.

1. *You are not old enough until your parents say so.*
The Bible commands, "Children, obey your parents in the Lord, for this is right" (Ephesians 6:1). Because of their experience and knowledge, God can use parents to guide their children in their dating relationships. Parents do have the benefit of objectivity. The girl who asks this question should consider her parents' thoughts regarding her dating this older person.

2. *You are not old enough to date until you have read God's standards in Scripture for dating and will not compromise those standards.*
Many parents say that they won't allow their daughter to date until she is sixteen years old. I disagree. The question shouldn't revolve around chronological age, but rather maturity and responsibility. A sixteen-year-old girl may be no more emotionally mature than a twelve-year-old. Also, some sixteen-year-old girls are more mature than twenty-five-year-old women! I know some single adults in their thirties who shouldn't be dating! Really!

Readiness for dating depends upon one's values and the mature judgment to carry out those values. That is why I suggest that before dating begins, each teenager, especially the Christian teen, needs to study what the Bible teaches about sex and dating. Then determine to live by those principles.

3. *You are not old enough to date until you understand your sexuality.*
Far too many teenagers learn about sex through the Braille system. Blindly touching and tasting sex can be very destructive. Your sexual knowledge should come from your parents, pastor, or youth counselor. It should not be the result of *Teen* magazine, slumber-party stories under the sheets, and trial-and-error experiences in dating. Somewhere young men and women should have the basics about sex before dating habits are formed. The tragic statistics of teenage pregnancies, abortions, and venereal disease testify to the glaring ignorance of America's "enlightened" youth culture.

4. *You are not old enough to date until you understand the main purpose of dating.*
Contrary to popular opinion, the main purpose of dating is not to practice your sex technique. Dating is not lab work, where we develop our skills in petting, and so forth.

The main purpose of dating is to develop close and intimate friendships. Developing real friendships demands maturity. Spiritual oneness can only happen when two people act responsibly toward each other. Dating is the door to friendship, then, later, courtship.

### *Too Old, Too Young*

Now, having laid this groundwork, we're ready to answer this question of dating people of differing ages. If two people meet the four qualifications we've mentioned, the actual age makes very little difference in most cases. Of course, a forty-year-old man dating a sixteen-year-old girl leaves something to be desired. Yet when that same girl is thirty years old and the man is now fifty-four, very few people would object to their romance and even marriage. So you see, age is relative to other factors. An eighteen-year-old boy dating a twenty-eight-year-old woman would seem very strange, but when he is a bit older—say twenty-two—and she is thirty-two, they seem more compatible. Each couple will have to weigh the variables and consult those concerned (parents and family), then seek God's guidance in these matters.

*He who sleeps with dogs*
*arises with fleas.*
*He who runs with the wolf*
*soon learns to howl.*

# 7 What Do You Think About "Missionary" Dating?

**I'VE HEARD IT SAID THAT A CHRISTIAN SHOULD NOT DATE OR MARRY A NON-CHRISTIAN, BUT HOW ARE YOU GOING TO WITNESS TO NON-CHRISTIANS IF YOU DON'T DATE THEM? CAN'T DATING BE USED TO SHARE CHRIST?**

This question addresses itself to what is known as "missionary dating." I've always smiled at that phrase. I've never dated a missionary, nor have I seen many missionaries dating! Anyway, I know what they mean. Can a Christian use his or her date as a means of winning others to Christ? I'm inclined to answer with a direct *yes,* but my experience tells me it's not that simple. Have you noticed that the really important things in life are always more complicated than we'd like them to be?

### *Unequally Yoked*

In 2 Corinthians 6:14, the apostle Paul warns us "Do not be bound together with unbelievers; for what partnership have righteousness and lawlessness, or what fellowship has light with darkness?" Good question, Paul! And the answer is obvious: little or none. We, as believers, truly are "unequally yoked" with nonbelievers in almost every area of life. It seems clear to me that Scripture here and elsewhere forbids the Christian to marry a non-Christian. This would also give guidance regarding serious dating. Yet, is there *ever* a time for dating an unbeliever in order to influence him for Christ? (For a full discussion of this subject, see chapter 11 "Can a Christian Date or Marry a Non-Christian?" in the author's book *Questions New Christians Ask.*)

### *Good But Risky*

Here my advice must be very guarded because some young reader may misunderstand this counsel. Yes, Christians can spend "boy-girl" time together regardless of their religion or lack of it. However, "dating," by my own definition (*see* chapter 1) is reserved for very special close friendships between two *Christians.* This does not mean that a Christian guy cannot spend time together with a non-Christian girl. When I was a fifteen-year-old boy, I started going to church with a pretty Christian girl. I was not a Christian at the time, had no interest in religion, but I went to church to be with her. My motives were shallow, but God used my attraction to her to win me to Himself. However, it doesn't always work that way. Sometimes the Christian gets too emotionally involved with the lost person and can be led astray. It goes both ways. I remember a few years ago an outstanding athlete at Texas Tech University came to my office to tell me he was going to do missionary work with a cheerleader. This fine Christian ball player found out a month later that he was becoming the *converted* rather than the *converter!* He told me, "Man, she started leading me instead of me leading her. Her morals are terrible, and I realized I couldn't handle the temptation." This guy had to act like Joseph running from Potiphar's wife!

### *Keep It Casual and Crowded*

My advice is that if you are going to use date time to witness, you'd best keep the relationship "friendly" but not romantic. Tell yourself and the other person your intentions with no pretense of courtship. Also, keep it casual and crowded. That is, go to group things, church functions, and so forth, and avoid being paired off in risky circumstances. It is wrong to lead someone on sexually when your motives are supposedly only to witness. No one likes to be a prospect for your religion. If you have a real interest in the lost person, develop a genuine caring friendship, but keep it on a nondating level. Then heed the advice of Scripture to "Watch over your heart with all diligence, For from it flow the springs of life" (Proverbs 4:23). You never know whom you'll fall in love with!

# 8 If Two Unsaved People Marry, and One Becomes a Christian, But Not the Other, Should They Divorce?

**MY PARENTS WERE HAPPILY MARRIED, UNTIL MY MOTHER BECAME VERY RELIGIOUS. SHE HAS BECOME A "BORN-AGAIN" CHRISTIAN AS SHE CALLS HERSELF. SINCE THIS HAS HAPPENED TO HER, SHE AND MY FATHER FIGHT A LOT. MOTHER IS TALKING ABOUT GETTING A DIVORCE. IS THIS RIGHT?**

What a sad situation. When Christ comes into a family, He desires to come as a healer and helper. This is not always the case. Like the question before us, I've known of cases where a husband or wife comes to Christ only to find that Jesus did not bring peace but a sword (Matthew 10:34–36). Yet, Jesus is not always responsible for the strife religion causes. Most of the time overly zealous religious people misunderstand what Christ teaches and misinterpret it to their marriage partner. Should a "saved" wife divorce her "unsaved" husband? No. The apostle Paul gives some very direct counsel on this situation:

> But to the rest I say, not the Lord, that if any brother has a wife who is an unbeliever, and she consents to live with him, let him not send her away.

And a woman who has an unbelieving husband, and he consents to live with her, let her not send her husband away.

For the unbelieving husband is sanctified through his wife, and the unbelieving wife is sanctified through her believing husband; for otherwise your children are unclean, but now they are holy.

Yet if the unbelieving one leaves, let him leave; the brother or the sister is not under bondage in such cases, but God has called us to peace.

For how do you know, O wife, whether you will save your husband? Or how do you know, O husband, whether you will save your wife?

1 Corinthians 7:12–16

You can't get an answer any more explicit than this. Paul says that the new Christian wife is to be a positive influence on her unbelieving husband. She's to make a believer out of him! This can and will happen, when she shows the love of God through her love for the husband. In fact, because she is now a Christian, she ought to be a *better* wife. Her religion ought to make her a more attractive person than she's ever been.

### *Conflicts—Yes; Divorce—No*

This does not mean that there might not be conflicts between them. I know a couple who used to go nightclubbing every Saturday night to dance and drink. When the wife became a Christian, she lost the desire for the nightlife. She told her husband she didn't want to go any more. He became very angry and started going without her. She came to me for counseling. I suggested that she offer him some creative alternatives. She did, and she eventually led her man to Christ. She could have condemned him as a rotten sinner—and lost him and her marriage. Instead he was attracted to her love, sincerity, and devotion to him.

***The Children, Too***

Notice that the Bible says that the believing wife "sanctifies" the children too (v. 14). She becomes an influence for good in the lives of her children. God promises to bless her children through her faithfulness. Even if her husband leaves, God will build a hedge about her for protection.

# 9 Is It All Right for a Girl to Phone a Guy?

**MY MOM SAYS A GIRL SHOULD NOT BE PUSHY WITH BOYS, LIKE ASKING THEM FOR DATES OR EVEN CALL A BOY ON THE PHONE. WHAT DO YOU THINK: IS IT ALL RIGHT FOR A GIRL TO PHONE A GUY?**

This question sounds like an Ann Landers-Dear Abby type question. It even sounds a little silly to some of us "old pros." Right? Yet, it is a good question. What is a girl's role in seeking a date? Should she wait till called or should she be the caller rather than the callee?

### *The Phone*

Every teenager has learned to use the phone. It is *the* source of communication. I live in a house with four kids and believe me, our phone rings constantly. Maybe it's not true, but it seems that girls like to talk on the phone more than guys. Maybe girls just talk more—period! Probably not, but it seems that way. Girls call girls, guys call guys, guys call girls. But should girls call guys—that's the question. Sometimes it's okay. If a girl has a boyfriend (in the sense of *friend*) and it is really a friendship, she has every right to call him up just to talk.

### *Pushy Piggy*

However, if a girl calls lots of guys on the phone and her motive is to flirt and try to get something started, then I'd say definitely not. I'm a disc jockey in my city, and you'd be amazed at the girls who call D.J.s to flirt with them on the phone. It's obscene! The Bible describes an aggressive and flirty female: "A beautiful woman lacking discretion and modesty is like a fine gold ring in a pig's snout" (Proverbs 11:22 TLB). That's a funny verse! It's also a very accurate description of a "forward" girl.

### *Play It Cool*

Most of us seem to want what we can't have, or what's hard to get. Girls, remember that. If you want a guy to notice you, don't come on too strong. Calling him up makes you look too "easy," perhaps even cheap. There are other, more subtle ways to get his attention. Calling up a guy should be reserved for the time when he is already *your* guy, or else he is a good friend.

# 10 What Is Flirting?

**WHAT IS FLIRTING? MY MOTHER SAYS A GIRL SHOULDN'T FLIRT, BUT I'M NOT SURE WHAT SHE MEANS. I'VE ASKED HER, AND ALL SHE SAYS IS, "YOU KNOW WHAT I MEAN." WELL, I DON'T, AND BESIDES, WHY CAN'T A GIRL FLIRT IF A BOY CAN?**

*Webster's Dictionary* defines flirting as "making insincere advances, to play at love without serious intentions." I agree, yet there is more involved than that. Why does your mother warn you against flirting? She obviously feels it is not in your best interest. As a father, I don't want my daughter "making insincere advances" to young men. Why? Okay, since you asked, I'll tell you.

### *Young and Naive*

Younger teenage girls are often naive about flirting. One may make it known to a boy that she likes him in many obvious ways. She uses "body language"—a look, a smile, a wink, or whatever it takes. She writes him notes, calls him on the phone, tells a girl friend to tell the guy she likes him. All of this is very innocent and a part of growing up. I don't attack such behavior except to say we need to outgrow it as a means of communication, mainly because flirting, which is cute in early teens, becomes improper behavior in maturing young women later on. To me, flirting is defined as using sexual language to attract attention. It is saying to a person of the opposite sex, "I'm attracted to you and I want you to like me, so I'm baiting the hook with sexual advances." When a girl uses her physical "attributes" to bait a guy she has already established the relationship on a sexual/physical level. She's giving off strong vibes. Far too often girls do this, turning on a guy only to discover they can't turn him off! She threw her meat to the hungry male lion, and now he's come to eat her up. Don't be naive, girls. When you flirt with guys, they are getting the message loud and clear. Is it the message you want them to hear from you? Only you can decide.

### *Leading Them On*

I've had guys say to me, "What's with these chicks? They flirt, tease, and urge you on, then when you start to make out, they'll say, 'What kind of girl do you think I am?' " Young lady, if you're not prepared to cook, don't light the fire! Leading guys on isn't wise, Christian, or ladylike. It can get you into trouble or give you a reputation you don't want.

### *What About the Guys?*

Flirting sexually can be done by the guys as well as girls. There is a difference between being friendly, winsome, or outgoing—and flirting. Flirting says, "I'm available to you in other ways than just friends." It seems to me we ought to develop friendships first and not separate our sexuality as a "product" we're advertising on the open market. What both guys and gals need to understand is that we're not to separate the body from the spirit. You are not a body with a spirit or a spirit with a body. You are a united self—a person. Therefore, girls, if you are flirtatious with a guy, he often thinks you are *inside* what you are showing him on the *outside*. Many times he's right. That's why God says, "Be beautiful inside, in your hearts, with the lasting charm of a gentle and quiet spirit which is so precious to God" (1 Peter 3:4 TLB).

### *Getting His Attention*

You may be really mad at me right now. I hope not, but if so, let me show you some other ways to get your man without flirting. That's right, there is another and better way. Scott Kirby, in his little book *Dating* (Baker House) makes some good suggestions on pages 67, 68 on how to attract a guy's attention discreetly. Let me share some of his thoughts and add a few of my own.

1. *Understand the shyness of most males.*
Some guys want to ask you out but fear rejection. Sometimes he needs a signal from you that you are interested.
2. *Use the light in your eyes.*
Nothing speaks louder in your female arsenal than your eyes. That's right—your eyes. Get his attention and give him that special "look." You know, the look that says, "I think you are wonderful; please ask me out." (Of course you could overdo it, right?)
3. *Be an attentive listener.*
Men are vain; they love to be listened to by women they admire. By your sincere interest you'll make him feel he's a king, and his opinion really counts.
4. *Get a friend to help you.*
Sometimes a mutual friend can tell (ever so discreetly) your guy that you might be interested in going out with him. Of course, if your friend isn't discreet, you may be worse off!
5. *Double dates are a start.*
My first date with my wife was arranged like this: My roommate's girl friend "arranged" for us to tag along in order to get us together. It worked! Besides, double dates are often the best way to get acquainted, especially if you are with neat friends who are fun to be with. It can take some of the awkwardness out of the first date.
6. *Share the same interests and activities.*
Be at the same parties or social gatherings. That gives you an opportunity to get to know him casually. Be careful not to come on

too strong. You don't want him to get the idea you are "chasing him." He needs to chase *you* (he thinks) until *you* catch him!

7. *Ask God: Counsel and help.*

God is interested in whom you date and develop friendships with. Pray about it. If nothing develops, don't force it (flirting) but accept it as God's will and move on to other things.

# 11 Should You Kiss on a First Date?

**SHOULD YOU ALLOW A KISS ON A FIRST DATE? MANY OF MY FRIENDS DO, BUT SOME DON'T. WE'RE ALL CONFUSED ABOUT IT. WHAT'S A GOOD RULE OF THUMB?**

Here's a neat question. Well, for a rule of thumb, don't use your thumb! If you do, there may not be a second kiss! The reason I say it's a neat question is because it's an almost obsolete question. In our permissive society where sex is easy, it's refreshing to find teenagers who are concerned about such things as kissing! Many are already on the Pill; they moved beyond kissing ages ago!

### *What Surveys Tell Us*

In 1980, *Seventeen* magazine (March 1980) surveyed one thousand teenage girls from all across America for the article "What You Want Out of Life." Various questions were asked. Among them was "How do you feel about pre-marital sex and living together before marriage?" On the question of pre-marital sex, 43 percent (430 out of 1,000 girls) said there is nothing wrong with it, and they intend to try it or have done it. This figure (43 percent) jumps to 60 percent among the 18- to 19-year-old girls. On the question of living together before marriage 36 percent see nothing wrong with it. So you see, kissing on a first date is hardly an issue with many girls today.

However, don't be misled by surveys. A survey can only tell you what everybody's doing. It cannot tell you what everyone *ought* to be doing. There is a difference. Surveys only *reflect* cultural values; they do not determine values.

### *What Is a Kiss, Anyway?*

To some young people, a kiss is no more meaningful than a handshake. It's casual, common, and uneventful. To others a kiss is very special and full of meaning and portent. Some make too little of it; others make too much out of it. Of course, kisses come in different shapes and sizes. There are long kisses and short kisses. There are passionate kisses and friendly kisses. There are dry kisses and juicy (ugh) kisses! The Bible even speaks of holy kisses (Thessalonians 5:26). Now, a holy kiss doesn't mean kissing in church on the back row! A holy kiss has to do with the reason for kissing. There are some noble and honorable reasons for a kiss. God is not against a good kiss. He's all for it, when it's *holy.*

### *Hearts and Lips*

What then is an honorable show of affection when kissing? When should it begin among two people? The first date? Maybe—just maybe—but not likely. Let me explain. A kiss to be meaningful and real should be the outward expression of the inward feeling of the heart. If all a boy feels for a girl is a casual friendship, then kisses should communicate the casualness of the relationship. What is dishonest is for two young people on a first date (or the tenth, for that matter), to make kissing a passionate TV love scene that does not represent their true feelings. A loving kiss can come out of a lying, lusting heart. A kiss that says, "I love you madly," just may mean, "I lust you badly."

Also, kissing is not a "game people play"—at least it shouldn't be. Kissing isn't practicing your sex technique. If you must practice, go kiss the mirror and make both of you sick! Really, where do we get the idea that kissing is *always* a part of dating? We didn't get that idea from God's Word. His Word tells us that our bodies are not for lust or immorality but to be used honorably. The Bible says, "God wants you to be holy and pure, and to keep clear of all sexual sin so that each of you will marry in holiness and honor—not in lustful passion as the heathen do, in their ignorance of God and his ways" (1 Thessalonians 4:3–5 TLB).

### *Kissing Not a Curse*

I don't mean to imply that kissing on a first date is a sin or that kissing itself is a curse. What is needed is for each of us to evaluate the kind of dating relationships we think God wants us to have. Then behave accordingly. There is a time and place for a physical show of affection. I know a pastor who kisses all the women in his church—regardless of their age. He "salutes" them with a "holy kiss." It's very beautiful.

So, whatever you decide, don't act under compulsion to "prove something." You don't *have* to kiss on the first or any date. Kissing doesn't make you mature, cool, or even a great lover. Being honest, open, and really caring makes you a neat person to be with.

# 12 Is French Kissing a Sin?

Now, here's a loaded question. I want to reply I've never kissed a Frenchman and I don't speak French. However, I won't do that. I'll play the role of counselor rather than comic. French kissing, right or wrong? Okay, as almost everybody knows, a "French" kiss as it is known, is a "wet one." It's a tongue-in-mouth kind of thing. No, not your mouth—someone else's! Sounds rather crude when you describe it, doesn't it? Many things in life that seem very beautiful at the time look so ugly under the microscope.

French kissing, that passionate display of great desire, brings mixed emotions from people. I often speak to sorority groups and discuss this subject of French kissing with college women. They either hate it or love it. Most all prefer to save it for that special guy. French kissing is definitely not on their list for good-night kisses or a casual date. Nearly all agree French kissing with someone you care for is a very exciting, erotic experience. I wonder why?

### *What M&J Have to Say*

I found out why French kissing is so much of a "turn on" with the right person. Doctors Masters and Johnson explained it in one of their sexy books (yes, all their books are about sex). Doctors M&J are sex therapists. In laboratory experiments they made some startling observations about French kissing as "foreplay" in sexual arousal. These skilled therapists say that French kissing is not an innocent "fun" way to kiss. They say it is an acting out of sexual intercourse in a very graphic way.

The tongue and mouth are "substitute" sex organs. The cigarette smoker uses the cigarette as a pacifier; French kissing is playacting at sexual intercourse. Masters and Johnson observed that the tongue is like the male penis, the mouth the female vagina. The thrusting in and out simulates the real thing. French kissing then becomes *the* most intimate of sexual experiences exceeded *only* by sexual intercourse. It is not child's play and innocent petting. It is more like dynamite than a firecracker.

### ***Lighting the Fires of Passion***

What all this means is that French kissing really is "foreplay," preparation for intercourse. French kissing definitely lights the fires of passion. I don't recommend it for casual dating. I don't recommend it for anyone who has problems controlling sexual arousal. It usually leads to other things that are lustful and therefore sinful. 'Nuf said!

# 13 What About Public Display of Affection?

**WHAT DO YOU THINK ABOUT COUPLES PETTING IN A P.D.O.A. (PUBLIC DISPLAY OF AFFECTION)? SOME OF MY FRIENDS ALMOST "MAKE OUT" IN CHURCH. I THINK IT'S DISGUSTING. WHAT DO YOU THINK?**

I think I probably agree with you! I agreed with you when I was a teenager. Most of the guys I ran around with thought it was sissy to "hang away" on your girl in public. That didn't mean we were all that pure in dark secret places! We just didn't do it in public. There is even some honor among thieves, I guess. I've asked thousands of teenagers in our seminars to vote by a show of hands on what they feel about "P.D.O.A." Always they overwhelmingly disapprove of it, especially the older, more mature teenagers. P.D.O.A. such as kissing, hugging, and so forth, is more a problem among younger teens than older. It is certainly a mark of immaturity. More than that, it is a mark of poor upbringing. It reflects a rudeness that does not consider the feelings of others who have to watch the "mating" going on. Sex at its best is a very private thing, and at its worst it is made cheap by going public. Teenagers by the hundreds have told me that they feel P.D.O.A. makes a girl seem cheap. They wonder, *If they behave this way in public, what do you suppose they do when they are alone?* Good question.

***Holding Hands and Other Things***

The question may arise, "What kind of touching and physical affection is appropriate in public?" Should a girl allow a guy to put his arm around her waist? Hold hands? Should she put her arm around him? Is a quick, polite kiss okay? Again, I don't have any concrete yes-or-no answers. It comes down to motive again. Do you want Christ to be honored by your witness? Are you aware that your body belongs to the Lord (not your boy or girl friend)? Does your physical affection represent the true character of your relationship? There is a great deal of difference between a college-age couple who are engaged showing some moderate affection like arms around each other, than, say, a junior-high couple doing the same thing. The physical affection should be an honest expression of the deep love and commitment. It should exist *private* or public in casual relationships. Which brings me to my real point. Sex should not be casual! When it's on display, it *is* casual. It looks casual and reflects bad judgment. Both guys and girls need to remember this and stay clear of those who treat sex, kissing, stroking, and such as a casual experience like shaking hands. It's just not the same, is it?

*The girl who uses her body as bait*
*to catch and keep her guy,*
*just may catch a flesh-eating shark—*
*Jaws I and II*

# 14 Can Sexy Clothes Be a "Turn On" That Displeases God?

**I AM A HIGH-SCHOOL SENIOR AND I'M DATING A REALLY NICE CHRISTIAN GIRL. YET, SHE HAS THIS PROBLEM WITH THE CLOTHES SHE WEARS. MAYBE I'M THE ONE WHO HAS THE PROBLEM. SHE WEARS THESE REALLY SEXY DRESSES AND TIGHT-FITTING CLOTHES. IS IT WRONG FOR A GIRL TO DRESS THAT WAY? HOW CAN I TELL HER IT BOTHERS ME? I SOMETIMES THINK SHE DOES IT BECAUSE SHE KNOWS IT BOTHERS ME.**

Confessions of an honest soul. I thought I was the only male whose eyes looked elsewhere before looking at her face. Yes, my friend, we can sin against others by the immoral suggestive clothes we wear (or don't wear). Both guys and gals need to be aware that clothes can be a means of *defrauding* others (*see* Glossary).

### *What You See Is What You Get*

In fact, I think most of us *know* what we're doing when we dress improperly. When a girl dresses sensually, she *knows* it. So does the young man who unbuttons the top two buttons of his shirt to reveal *both* hairs on his chest!

God has a word for us about dressing improperly. Proverbs 7:10 warns young men to beware of the woman "dressed as a harlot." You and I know what the dress of a harlot looks like. She dresses so as to call attention to the tools of her trade. She wears clothing that reveals her thighs, hips, breasts, and so forth. She is on display. She wants you to notice the wrapper (her body). She cares little about you liking her (spirit) personally.

What is shameful is that too often Christian girls dress this way. Sometimes even without thinking about it. Frequently we wear what's *in* rather than what's decent and proper. Girls, you can turn guys on by the way you display your body. Your clothing can become a cause of stumbling (*see* Romans 14:13,21) to men. Men can do the same to women by the clothing they wear.

### *Fig Leaves and Other Fashions*

Before we discuss what is proper to wear, we should think about the purpose of clothing in the beginning. Why did God clothe Adam and Eve?

They were originally nude, without notice or need of clothing. In fact, there was no such thing as clothing. There was no necessity for it. The first couple, in their innocence, knew nothing of nakedness. Lusting was not a part of their existence. Then came the Fall. After Adam and Eve sinned, their entire inner nature was affected (and ours also as a result). Now they had hearts capable of lust. God knew this, and told them to cover themselves. Their fig leaves were mute testimony to their sinfulness. Clothing was commanded by God the Father for a twofold purpose. First, a covering to prevent runaway lust. Clothes are for a covering. They are meant to cover the body and its sexual parts. Remember this the next time you buy clothes. They are not to make you more sexy, but to make you *less* sexy. They are to limit lust, not create it. Second, clothes were for protection. Adam and Eve lived in a perfect environment before the Fall. After they were expelled from Eden, there was a need for protective clothing. (After the flood, there would be a whole new world of changing climate. Before the flood, the earth was probably tropical throughout. *See The Genesis Flood,* John C. Whitcomb and H. M. Morris.) These two simple purposes should guide us in the purchase of clothing. Clothes do not have to be an adornment like jewels to call attention to us. It is one thing to look nice and quite another thing to look like a display dummy.

### *Look Into My Eyes*

I have a wise word to you girls about dress fashions. When you dress up, realize the most wonderful thing about you is your spirit (it *should* be). I realize a boy can't *see* your spirit, or can he? Yes, he can. By looking into your eyes he can see the real you. Your personality shines out through your eyes. You should dress in order to call attention to your eyes—not your body. If a boy looks at you and never looks above your neck, you've dressed wrongly. He shouldn't be tempted to do a "body check" before he looks at your face and says, "Hi." Don't tempt him that way. How do you get his attention to look into your eyes so you can hypnotize him with your spell? I hate to mention this but the Bible says your hair is your secret weapon. That's right, your hair is your *glory.* That's what the Bible says in 1 Corinthians 11:15. Why is this true? Because your hair, ladies, is the "frame" for your face. If your hair is beautiful, it calls attention to your face, and the focal point of your face is your eyes! Therefore, to get a man to notice you (the real you), give diligence to your hair and your eyes. Your clothing should not detract from your face. Clothing fashions do not have to dictate how you will dress. A girl should decide what looks fashionable on her, and dress accordingly. There are certain classic fashions that are always in and are proper and elegant.

### *Swimsuits and Suntans*

Perhaps I'm really meddling here, but swimsuits on both men and women are a good example of where the Christian must use some judgment. Most swimsuits for women today just are not decent for a Christian to wear. With a little effort, you can find a suit that doesn't defraud the guys. The same advice is applicable to the men. Remember, first impressions are important, and people judge us by our appearance. As ambassadors for Christ, we represent the King of kings—dress accordingly.

# 15 What If Your Christian Boyfriend Wants to Have Sex and You Don't?

**I AM SIXTEEN YEARS OLD. MY BOYFRIEND AND I ARE BOTH CHRISTIANS. WE GREW UP IN THE SAME CHURCH AND OUR FAMILIES ARE CLOSE FRIENDS. WE'VE BEEN DATING FOR ABOUT A YEAR. MY BOYFRIEND IS EIGHTEEN AND VERY MATURE. WE'VE HAD PROBLEMS WITH SEX, BUT I'M STILL A VIRGIN. MY PROBLEM IS THAT HE WANTS TO "GO ALL THE WAY" AND I DON'T. I REALLY CARE FOR HIM, BUT HE'S REALLY BUGGING ME ABOUT THIS. WHAT CAN I DO?**

Here we have two very different responses to sexual urges. A young woman under control and her guy out of control. He no doubt cries out, "I just can't help myself," while she in turn thinks he *can* and *should* control himself. She thinks he should behave like a Christian, and he thinks he needs sex to show his love for her. He says, "If you love me, you will have sex with me," and her response is, "If you loved me, you wouldn't ask me to disobey God!" They for sure have a conflict. Their problem is so common, even among churchgoing teens, that I wanted to include it in this section of the book.

### *Needs and Wants*

First of all, sex *is* a real genuine need. The desires are really there—just like the desire for water or food. Sex can be a physical craving—yet unlike the need for water or food, you won't die if you don't get it. One can fast for a time sexually, just as you can fast for a time where food or water is concerned. All our physical cravings seem to go through cycles. This is pointed out by John White in his book *Eros Defiled,* when he observes that these cravings or desires come in phases.

*Preliminary Phase*

Sex, like any other physical need, begins in restlessness, or a mild desire, say to drink, or eat.

*Phase I*

The second stage of desire is agitation, or an intense thirst, hunger, or feeling for the need to be fulfilled.

*Phase II*

Next comes alleviation, the satisfying of that need, through drinking, or eating.

*Phase III*

Relaxation and relief follow the loss of desire, which has been satisfied.

These patterns of anxiety and satisfaction apply to sexual desire. Something happens to create restlessness (petting, a pretty girl, a book, a movie), then comes agitation or arousal. At this point we can either continue the agitation and even seek alleviation, or we can *remove* that which caused the restlessness and agitation. This is true in dating and physical sexual arousal. Our sexual urges are not continual, steady things. They come and go. When a desire reaches intense agitation, God can and will make provision for "unbearable" urges like sex. Everyone can testify that urges can be controlled—even put off. A child may be starving one minute, then when his favorite television show comes on, you can't get him to the dinner table. His interests have been shifted. The same is true of sex. Neither hunger for food nor hunger for sex increase automatically, until we explode into uncontrollable behavior. Sexual desire is like a spring in an alarm clock, wound up tightly until ready for release. And should that release not come, you need feel no real discomfort.

### *I Can't Help Myself*

Therefore, when your boyfriend (or girl friend) says in that moment of utmost agitation (Phase I), "I've just got to have sex; I just can't help myself," we need to understand that this is just not the case. It is not true. You can and should control yourself. By redirecting your interest elsewhere (find a television program), your hunger can wait.

### *Shape Up or Ship Out*

If your boyfriend can't straighten up his act, you should tell him the act is over—shape up or ship out. Such uncontrollable behavior is a mark of immaturity. Of course, if you, young lady, are the cause of his agitation, *you* should shape up. Perhaps you "rev up" his engine, then try to cut him off. It's your decision—make a good one.

*True friends like ivy and the wall*
*stand together or fall together.*

*Thomas Carlyle*

# 16 How Can I Help a Friend Who Has Had Sexual Problems?

**HOW CAN I HELP A FRIEND WHO HAS BEEN IN TROUBLE SEXUALLY? I KNOW A GIRL WHO CONTINUALLY GETS MESSED UP WITH GUYS. WHAT CAN I SAY TO HER?**

The girl who continually gets messed up sexually is very fortunate to have a friend who cares about her. If you are a girl, you can relate to her much better than a guy could. You women understand each other.

Far too often a girl gets a bad reputation from her loud-mouthed boy "friends" who messed around with her under the guise of "making love." Living down a bad reputation isn't easy. It's easier to get one than to get rid of it. A girl with a bad reputation sexually sometimes reacts by becoming even more rebellious. She talks an"I'll show you how bad I can be" attitude. A girl like that needs a true friend who doesn't judge her but tries to understand her and challenge her to change her life-style.

## *Angels and Demons*

What I've discovered is that most bad girls aren't really all that bad. Immoral sex may tarnish but it need not destroy. These "loose" girls were once pure and can be pure again by God's grace. It's not a big step from angel to demon. Actually, devils were once angels—right?

The best way to help a girl who seems to go from one sordid affair to another is pray for her, first of all. Ask God to work in her heart. James says, ". . . The earnest prayer of a righteous man has great power and wonderful results" (James 5:16 TLB). Second, become her friend. Accept her as she is. Let her know that even though you don't approve of her behavior, you still accept and love her. Third, seek to surround her with Christian friends, to get her away from so much dependence upon boyfriends. If she finds the love she needs among girl friends, she'll not lean so heavily on her guy. Then, share God's love with her. Get her to read His Word. Appeal to her spirit through Scripture that points out her impurity as well as God's forgiveness. Such verses as Ephesians 5:3 are good: "But do not let immorality or any impurity or greed ever be named among you, as is proper among saints." Get her to face the challenge of Scripture. Her great need may be to become a child of God. Once she knows Jesus, His Spirit in her can do "office work" to rearrange her values. Remember, *you* can't reform a lost person. She needs to be transformed by the new birth Jesus talked about.

### *Seventy Times Seven*

I once knew a prostitute I met on Sunset Strip in Hollywood, California. After many weeks of listening to this eighteen-year-old girl, I finally led her to Christ. However, she did not change overnight. Her old sexual patterns continued for some time. My heart saddened, as she would tell me she had "slipped" again. However, I remained her friend, tried not to judge her, just love her in Christ. Finally she came through for the Lord and herself. Later she told me, "Barry, if you hadn't stood by me, I couldn't have made it. Thank you for not quitting on me." That's what it takes, forgiving "seventy times seven." It is a real struggle, but such friendship often pays off in changed lives.

*Youth is a time of change.*
*They say between the ages of thirteen to eighteen*
*a parent can age thirty years.*

# 17 What Role Should Parents Play in My Dating Plans?

**I'VE HEARD IT SAID THAT A GUY SHOULD TALK TO THE FATHER OF THE GIRL ABOUT ASKING HER OUT FOR A DATE. IS THIS A GOOD POLICY? WHAT ROLE SHOULD PARENTS PLAY IN DATING? WHAT IF THEY DON'T CARE WHAT YOU DO? WHAT IF THE PARENTS AREN'T CHRISTIANS?**

Boy, am I glad someone asked this question. I'm glad because most teenagers want and need their parents' advice. Amazingly, today's youth feel that their parents' opinions are more important to them than the opinions of their peers. In the *Seventeen* magazine article mentioned earlier, "What You Want Out of Life," one thousand girls surveyed revealed that a majority of them value highly their parents' opinion. That's surprising to many people, especially teenagers. There's the so-called generation gap we all hear about. It's true, it exists, but kids need to hear what parents have learned from past experiences.

### *My Parent—The Jerk*

Advising kids to involve their parents seems absurd to lots of teenagers. However, I have my reasons for suggesting it. First of all, parents have the benefit of experience about dating. They just may not be the jerks you think they are. You can learn from their experience. I bet your mom was a real cool chick in her day! Why make mistakes when you can avoid them and have a better time? Why does each generation of youth have to bloody their noses on the same bad trip that the previous generation did? A wise man learns from history, even his parents' history. Also, your parents should be involved in your date life because they have the benefit of objectivity. You can't see your boyfriend through the same eyes that your mother can, girls. Fella, your dad isn't lovesick over that girl as you are. He can be more objective about her than you can. He sees a wart on the nose as a wart on the nose, not just a blemish that makeup can hide. So, yes, your parents can give counsel regarding your dating.

### *Ask My Daddy*

Should a guy ask the girl's father for permission to date? Not a bad idea in most cases. It can really help you girls. When Charlie Creep calls on the phone and asks you out, let ol' Dad bail you out. Tell Charlie, "I have to ask my dad; can you wait just a moment?" Then with your hand over the mouthpiece you tell Dad, "Charlie Creep wants to take me out. Please say no, so I don't have to go with him." See—Dad can take all the blame and you get off the hook! I'm just kidding, but it does work that way at times. My teenage girl will work it that way when she starts dating.

### *Treat Her Like a Queen*

I suggest even that a father should take his daughter out for her first date. Dad can show her a great time, treat her like a lady, and show daughter how it's supposed to be done. I promise you, Dad, she'll never forget it. Also, every guy from now on will have to measure up to her dad! Not a bad idea. I'm going to do just that with my girl next year. You can ask her some day how it went!

### *My Parents Don't Care*

Some of you have parents who aren't Christians, or parents who just refuse to take an interest in your date life for one reason or another. What do you do then? Okay, if parents will not guide you with standards, why not seek help elsewhere? I did. When I was a teenager, my parents were divorced. I had no father to talk to. God provided leadership for me through my church. I had youth directors, Sunday-school teachers, and a pastor who met that need for me. Perhaps you can put yourself under the counsel of some mature Christian adult. Many times it's easier to talk to some other adult than it is to your own parents. There's nothing wrong with that. Just don't deliberately ignore your parents and hurt their feelings. (Yes, they *do* have feelings.)

At the risk of being nosy, parents need to ask appropriate questions from time to time to show the teenager that they are interested in their child's social life. This can encourage the teen to open up and share if he or she wants to. Also, parents should encourage their teenager to bring the "date" home from time to time to share dinner and family social time together. This helps everybody! Isolation brings death to parents and teens. Keep the lines of communication open—always.

# SEX

*Many teenagers are as confused about sex as a termite in a Yo-Yo!*

# 18 Is Thinking About Sex a Sin?

Proverbs says, "As a man thinks in his heart, so is he" (*see* 23:7). What this means is that all we are begins in what we think. My days are made up of thoughts. Someone said it this way:

*Sow a thought—you'll reap a deed.*
*Sow a deed—you'll reap a habit.*
*Sow a habit—you'll reap a character.*
*Sow a character—you'll reap a destiny.*

It is important that we guard our thoughts from evil. He who continually thinks evil becomes evil, and he who thinks good thoughts becomes a good person.

All of this brings up our next question. Is thinking about sex a sin? My answer—yes and no! How's that for evasiveness? I hedge because the question is more complicated than it appears.

### *It Is Common to Man*

Often young people tell me they feel dirty, or guilty, because they have many thoughts and daydreams about sex. They want to know if this is normal, or is it "weird" and sinful. To begin with, if you're weird for thinking about sex, my young friend, then welcome to a very weird world! A leading sociologist says the average teenage boy has sexual thoughts every twenty-nine seconds. I wonder if these thoughts increase or decrease with age?

What teenagers need to know first of all is that such thoughts are a normal part of their growing up. The teen years (and into early twenties) are peak years of sexual development. As the body develops, it produces sexual hormones at a rapid rate. The male reaches his sexual peak at ages seventeen or eighteen, according to Dr. Ed Wheat and his wife, Gaye, in their book *Intended for Pleasure.* So, teenager, your hormones are working overtime! It is natural that you experience an increased sexual awareness.

### *Where Did That Thought Come From?*

However, not all thoughts about sex are normal or good. To be sexually aware is one thing—but to be sexually obsessed is quite another matter. To look at a person of the opposite sex with admiration, even sexual attraction, is a very natural thing. But what about those thoughts that go beyond attraction to thoughts of imagined sexual activities with that person? You see, there is a fine line between looking and lusting. Remember Jesus warned us that looks can lead to lusting, and lusting is synonymous with adultery (Matthew 5:28). I remember years ago hearing Dr. Billy Graham saying in a sermon to young people that the first look isn't sin; it's the second look that can become sin. Perhaps that's what James was saying when he wrote, "But each one is tempted when he is carried away and enticed by his own lust" (James 1:14). We've already established that temptation itself is not sin—only yielding to it is sin. It has also been suggested by some Bible teachers that "thought" temptations can come from the evil one—Satan. Maybe those "fiery darts" thc apostle Paul says Satan shoots at us are evil thoughts he puts in our minds. If so, then we are faced with a decision about some sexual thoughts. If they are from Satan, they must be rejected, lest we cultivate them in lust. We must not be "enticed" and swallow the bait like a hungry fish.

***Fantasies and Daydreams***

Sexual thoughts become destructive when we allow them to run wild in our minds. A girl may think about a handsome boy with all his muscles and curly hair, but when she deliberately fantasizes about his making love to her, and so forth, she is then defrauding herself the same as if she were looking at a dirty magazine. Such thoughts create sexual arousal that cannot be righteously satisfied.

***This Mind in You***

Because we are what we think, we are challenged in Scripture to "Let this mind be in you, which was also in Christ Jesus" (Philippians 2:5 KJV). There are times when we must reject evil thoughts and ask Christ to give us His thoughts of purity and love for others. This He can and will do for those who are His children. He lives in the heart of the Believer and can live through his thoughts as well.

*Blessed are those*
*who know the difference between*
*their loving and their lusting,*
*for they shall be pure in heart*
*and understand the reason.*

*(from) Calvin Miller's*
*The Singer*

# 19 What Is Lust?

Jesus taught us that it is a sin to lust. He said, "You have heard that it was said, 'You shall not commit adultery'; but I say to you, that every one who looks on a woman to lust for her has committed adultery with her already in his heart" (Matthew 5:27,28). All right then, *what is lust? Are we all guilty of it from time to time? How can it be prevented?* These are commonly asked questions.

Most people I know would not admit to being adulterous. Yet all of us have experienced sexual lust. The dictionary defines lust as "sexual desire or appetite." This definition seems to imply that sexual desire or lust is evil or sinful. This is not true. Sexual desire is the gift of God. There is nothing evil in sexual desire itself. It's the misuse of that desire that can lead to sin. The New Testament word which Jesus used is the most common biblical word for lust. (The word in Greek is *epithumia,* from the word *thumos,* which means passion or longing. The preposition before the word *epi* gives it the idea of an "over" passion.) It means more than just "desire" for something. The word means a very strong passion. Lust is an *over*desire, or a passion out of control. Sexual arousal is normal, but uncontrolled, runaway sexual arousal is sinful and dangerous.

Most people feel no guilt consciousness or wrongdoing for lustful thoughts. To the average person, such thoughts are merely a normal part of everyday life. Jesus called it sin. He equated it with the actual physical act of adultery. The Bible illustrates graphically the tragic results of sexual lust in the lives of such men as Samson, David, and Solomon. Sexual lust is dishonoring to God and destructive to people. We need to learn to flee from it.

Is there a difference between temptation and lust? I think perhaps there is. It seems to me that lust is our response to temptation. In James, chapter 1, we read, "Let no one say when he is tempted, 'I am being tempted by God'; for God cannot be tempted by evil, and He Himself does not tempt any one. But each one is tempted when he is carried away and enticed by his own lust. Then when lust has conceived, it gives birth to sin; and when sin is accomplished, it brings forth death" (James 1:13–15). Here, then, is the pattern:

1. a temptation (stimulus)
2. sexual lust (response)
3. sexual sin (result)

This can be demonstrated rather easily. A man is walking past a newsstand. He glances at a magazine copy. There is a picture of a naked woman on the cover. His eyes see the picture. That is the moment of temptation. Now, temptation is not sinful; yielding to it *is* sinful. The man has a decision to make. He can look away and go on his way, or he can decide to go a step further. If he is "carried away and enticed by his own lust," he's in trouble spiritually. As he picks up the magazine and looks at its pornography, he is deliberately choosing to receive the temptation into his heart. The result is a lustful, adulterous act. He has sinned. So, by sexual lust, we mean any sexual thought or deed that is potentially disobedient or dishonoring to God and which is potentially degrading or destructive to people.

Make no mistake about it: all of us experience this struggle with sexual lust. We each face those situations, when we must choose whether to give in or to resist such temptation.

### *Walking With Your Eyes Closed*

How can we overcome sexual lust? In our sex-oriented society we face temptation many times each day. As one college man said to me, "I can't walk around with my eyes closed." Sexual temptation is real. For some it is more real than for others. To those of us who admit to the sin of sexual lust, we have a fight on our hands. We can't put on blinders or go join a monastery. What we can do is admit the problem and seek to deal with it through God's help. Also, we must not think that because we have lustful thoughts we are perverted or *over*sexed. The problem is common to all.

If you are not struggling with sexual lust, remember that lust may take many forms. Some lust for power, fame, wealth, or some other ego-gratifying pursuits. We are all tempted; we all experience failure. Remember, God has no favorite sinner. He has no favored sin. We are all in this struggle together. The best solution is to admit our failures, confess them to God who loves us, and try through His Spirit's power to restructure our lives. Be encouraged, God says: "No temptation has overtaken you but such as is common to man; and God is faithful, who will not allow you to be tempted beyond what you are able, but with the temptation will provide the way of escape also, that you may be able to endure it" (1 Corinthians 10:13). (*See* the next chapter "How Can I Control My Sexual Appetites?" Also, an excellent book on lust is *The Other Side of Love* by Mel White, Power Books, Revell.)

# 20 How Can I Control My Sexual Appetites?

God's Word challenges us when it declares, "But do not let immorality or any impurity or greed even be named among you, as is proper among saints" (Ephesians 5:3). When you are single and in your "prime," so to speak, it's not easy for some to remain pure sexually.

I often hear statements like this from couples: "But we love each other, and it's so hard to control our sex urges when we're together." These statements come from Christians, not Hugh Hefner pagans. Believers have hormones too—right? You bet we do!

Okay, how can our sexual desires be controlled so that we can live morally acceptable lives? A famous preacher, J. Wallace Hamilton, once compared our sexual desires to wild horses (in *Ride the Wild Horses*). Like wild horses, we can respond to sex one of three ways. Some suggest we let the horse run wild. This philosophy of free sex could be called *expressionism.* This approach says, "If it feels good, do it." Hugh Hefner, of *Playboy* magazine, has advocated free sex for years. The problem with such uncontrolled sex is that it is destructive to the individual, to the home, and to the nation. If you let the horse run wild, it will soon run over you! Without a doubt, expressionism is for "Gentiles who do not know God" (1 Thessalonians 4:5). A second response to our sexual appetites would be to "shoot the horse."

This attitude sees sex as either evil or only as a means of procreation. It certainly is not for pleasure—God forbid! This hush-hush sexual attitude could be called repression. Either way, a wild horse or a dead horse, we still have problems! Repression has never worked, nor will it. Trying to deny your sexual drives is much like putting a pail of water over a hot fire—it will eventually boil over, out of control. I guess if we could lock all the girls up in antique chastity belts (*see* Glossary), and chain up all the boys to fence posts, maybe we could keep them apart! Then again, I doubt it!

Scripture does *not* tell us that sex is evil. Sexual intercourse is neither a virtue nor a sin—in itself. The Word of God indicates that sex has a higher purpose than just to bring babies into the world. Sex has a purpose given in Scripture—to abolish isolation ("It is not good for the man to be alone . . ." Genesis 2:18, and *see* 2:23–25). Sex is God's gift to us to express intimacy, love, and commitment. It says, "I am yours alone, always." In the context of marriage, then, sex is good and not to be repressed or viewed as evil. For further reading on this subject *see* John White's *Eros Defiled, The Christian and Sexual Sin* (Intervarsity Press).

What then are we to do with this sometimes wild and uncontrollable horse called sexual desire? Let God ride the wild horses for you. Let His Holy Spirit control your sexual appetites. "Like a city that is broken into and without walls Is a man who has no control over his spirit" (Proverbs 25:28). The Christian needs to remember that self-control is a by-product of the Spirit-controlled life. Self-control is a fruit of the Spirit (Galatians 5:22). The Spirit of Christ in the Believer can empower him to live pure sexually.

It has always been an encouragement to me to know that Jesus Christ was tempted sexually also. The writer of Hebrews tells us that Jesus "has been tempted in all things as we are, yet without sin" (Hebrews 4:15). Did you catch that—"in all things"? That means Christ has been tempted sexually, but did not yield. He has ridden the wild horse, broken, tamed, and mastered it. He made it His servant. You and I need His power in us so we can do that!

***How to "Ride the Wild Horses"***

It seems the problem is not God's ability, but our inability to trust Him with our sexual desires. Far too many believers are overcome and overwhelmed by the lust of the flesh. What is needed is some instruction in how to trust Christ to deliver us. Then we need to decide to act upon this knowledge. God has not willed our defeat in the midst of any temptation. No Christian need ever say, "The devil made me do it," but God has always made a way of escape (1 Corinthians 10:13).

Are you aware that Satan's temptations only come in three areas of your life? He only has three bullets in his gun of temptation. This unholy trinity of temptation is found in 1 John 2:16, "For all that is in the world, the lust of the flesh and the lust of the eyes and the boastful pride of life, is not from the Father, but is from the world." Look closely at these three temptations:

*The lust of the flesh*—our physical desires
*The lust of the eyes*—our mental desires
*The pride of life*—our spiritual desires

Satan can tempt us only spiritually, mentally, or physically. These are the only weapons he has. Our sexual passions are one part of his area of attack. Yes, he even tempted Jesus in these areas. Matthew 4 records the great temptation of Christ. Satan fired all three bullets at our Savior and when the smoke cleared, Jesus stood victorious. Remember Satan came to Him after forty days and nights of fasting and tempted Jesus to turn the stones into bread. Just what was this temptation? Satan was saying, "God gave you physical appetites and He wants you to satisfy them." Has he ever tempted you like that? Sure he has! This appeal to the "lust of our flesh" is a common (even daily) temptation. How can we resist it?

I've heard this story many times. A teenage girl tells me she and her boyfriend are in love and having sex. She feels guilty about the sex, but she says that when they are together and begin to kiss, and so on, they just can't control themselves. She asks for help—what would you tell them to do? I tell them to do what Jesus did. He met this temptation and conquered it. He met it the same way you and I can meet it. He submitted His life and physical passions to God. The secret to riding those wild horses is not expressionism, or repression, but rather submission. We need to learn to submit them to God's control. We are given sound advice in James 4:7, 8: "Submit therefore to God. Resist the devil and he will flee from you. Draw near to God and He will draw near to you. . . ." This word *submit* is a military word. It means to be under the rule or command of someone. Jesus was under the authority of God and totally submitted. He was submitted to God in three areas:

*Jesus Was Submitted to the Word of God*

Our Lord quoted the Scriptures back to Satan at each temptation. He did so because He was totally submitted to the authority of God's Word. Now, you and I can quote Scripture to the devil when we are tempted. It's not a bad idea, but it won't change anything, unless we are submitted to God's Word. I've tried quoting verses to ward off temptation, and it doesn't work! It's not *quoting* it that works; it's *submitting* to it that works. Have you submitted your sexual desires to Scripture? Do you really believe what it says about your body and then act accordingly? When you do believe, and *daily* submit sexual needs to His Word, you'll begin to ride the wild horses.

*Jesus Was Submitted to the Will of God*

Satan again came to Jesus to tempt Him (Matthew 4:5–7). This time he appealed to lust of the eyes. He urged Jesus to cast Himself down from the top of the temple so all would see His miraculous rescue by mighty angels. Jesus again answered Satan with Scripture, "Ye shall not tempt the Lord your God . . ." (Deuteronomy 6:16 KJV). Think with me a minute. What was this temptation? It was an appeal to our Lord's desire to have His own way, to force God's hand. Listen, Satan will always try to dissatisfy you with the way God is running your life. The devil will always offer us shortcuts to success, fame, or happiness. Our sexual desires are an illustration of that. He says, "Why wait for marriage to have sex? You love each other; go ahead, it's all right."

You and I can overcome such appeals only if we, like our Lord Jesus, are submitted to God's will as well as God's Word. Jesus was committed to doing God's will, God's Way—are you? Do you really want His will done in your life? Satan has a rough time defeating those who know and love God's Word and desire earnestly to do God's will.

A high-school senior girl told me recently, "I'm a virgin; none of my friends are. They tease me a lot. It's hard to take, but I'd rather please God than my friends. That's what helps me most. I want Jesus to be pleased with me." That's it! She was submitted to God's will.

*Jesus Was Submitted to the Worship of God*

One last lesson to be learned from Christ's temptation—Satan offered Jesus all the kingdoms of this world if He would only worship him. Christ refused. He replied, "You shall worship the Lord your God, and serve Him only" (*see* Deuteronomy 6:13). You see, this is what Satan wanted all along. He wants to be worshiped. The devil has a God complex. Every temptation he brings our way is to lead us closer to worshiping him. Through our sin, he desires to control our lives. He can do that through our sexual desires. Only when we, like our Lord, desire to glorify and worship God with our bodies, will we ride the wild horses of sexual passion. We can, and we will do so when we are submitted to God's Word, will, and worship.

## Some Practical Helps

Some people have very little trouble with sexual lust; others fight the battle daily. Here are some practical words from Scripture to help you *submit:*

1. "Do not give the devil an opportunity" (Ephesians 4:27). Are you helping the devil out? By the sensual books you read—

movies you see—the places you go—are you continually arousing your sexual desires? In a dating relationship, do you create problems for yourself by being alone with your date in a tempting situation (the parked car, the living-room couch, and so on)?

2. "Abstain from all appearance of evil" (1 Thessalonians 5:22 KJV). Are the questionable sexual activities you are involved in petting, necking, making out? Do these activities "light the fires of passion" and turn on what's hard to turn off?

3. "Blessed is the man that endureth temptation: for when he is tried, he shall receive the crown of life . . ." (James 1:12 KJV). Think about the promise. A crown of life awaits you if you overcome sexual lust. Each moment, each day, each victory, you are being blessed. God is working His character in you.

4. "Thy word have I had in mine heart, that I might not sin against thee" (Psalms 119:11 KJV). When sexual temptation comes, have you committed to memory specific verses of Scripture that speak to your heart and rebuke the devil? If not, do so. By quoting the Word and submitting to it, you emulate the life of Christ and His victory.

5. ". . . pray, that ye enter not into temptation . . ." (Matthew 26:41 KJV). Have you trained to pray for victory before the fight begins? A couple who start their date with prayer are not likely to defraud each other sexually. Prayer puts God in the struggle with you. Pray and ride the wild horses!

6. ". . . better to marry than to burn" (1 Corinthians 7:9). Paul's advice to the unmarried is simple: "If they do not have self-control let them marry, for it is better to marry than to burn [with passion]." If a couple is in love, planning marriage, and can't control sexual passion, sometimes it is time to marry *now.*

# 21 How Do You Define Petting? Is It Wrong?

**MY GIRL FRIEND AND I REALLY LOVE EACH OTHER AND WE'RE BOTH CHRISTIANS. WE'VE SPENT A LOT OF TIME TOGETHER AND OFTEN WE START KISSING AND IT LEADS TO OTHER THINGS. HOW DO YOU DEFINE PETTING, AND IS IT WRONG?**

The Bible says through the apostle Paul, "It is good for a man not to touch a woman" (1 Corinthians 7:1). There's a verse that is certainly old-fashioned for today's fast-moving crowd! Don't even touch her, the Good Book says! Surely Paul didn't mean that! or did he? Whatever he meant, today's Christian singles are looking for some guidelines about sexual foreplay apart from "going all the way."

### *Petting and Other Things*

Ann Landers in one of her booklets for teens tries to make a distinction between "petting" and "necking." I read the booklet and laughed out loud! She says "necking" is kissing, hugging, caressing, and so forth. Petting is the heavier scene of touching sex organs, getting naked (all or partially), and bringing each other to a high sexual arousal or even climax without sexual intercourse. She implies that necking is okay and petting is a no-no! Here I think Miss Landers is either being silly, naive, or both! How can you draw the line and say necking is okay and petting is not okay? I agree completely with Dr. John White in *Eros Defiled,* when he says:

> How does one distinguish between petting and intercourse? Once you try to map out morality in terms of anatomy and physiology you wind up with an ethical labyrinth from which there is no exit.
>
> Take the example of a kiss. Can anyone take seriously a Roman Catholic writer who distinguished innocent kisses, venial sin kisses and mortal sin kisses by the number of seconds the lips touched? It is true that the further you proceed with physical contact the nearer you come to coitus. But defining coitus in terms of penetration and orgasm has as much moral significance and as much logical difficulty as trying to define a beard by the number of hairs on a chin.
>
> I know that experts used to distinguish light from heavy petting, and heavy petting from intercourse, but is there any moral difference between two naked people in bed petting to orgasm and another two having intercourse? Is the one act a fraction of an ounce less sinful than the other?
>
> Is it perhaps more righteous to pet with clothes on? If so, which is worse, to pet with clothes off or to have intercourse with clothes on?

That's a well-written, graphic section. What he is saying is that sexual foreplay and premarital intercourse are the same issue. They may sound and feel like different issues, but they are not. If penetration is wrong, then it seems to me fondling touches are also wrong. As a friend of mine says, "If you don't intend to cook, don't light the fire."

### *Guidelines or Guesses*

What I'm saying is, let's stop kidding ourselves about this "too far" business. Learning to behave honorably is not easy, and it will demand much self-control. Petting is for those who are immature, sensual, or both. It certainly is not wise, honorable, or spiritual. All I can say to this question is that a couple in love, promised or engaged, need to work out their own standards that leave them with a clear conscience and then stand by them. Each couple is different and will reach different conclusions. When kissing and caressing starts, some motive tests are helpful. Is your motive to get or to give? Are you a tease? Trying to show sweet affection and trying to turn on your partner are two very different motives. I offer no rules that say, "Thou shalt not kiss with your lips parted more than one-eighth of an inch, or thou shalt not kiss for more than ten seconds." What I do suggest is that you be honest with yourself and your date and that you "know thyself." Purpose to please God with your date life and follow the urges of your spirit, not your flesh, and you'll do all right.

Remember the question isn't "How far *are* we to go?" but rather, "How far *should* we go?" Go as far as real love will let you go honorably. That's God's way.

### *Unanswered Questions*

Of course, you're disappointed in my answer. What about French kissing, lying down together to kiss, or caressing other body parts, except breasts or genitals? You'll have to find those answers for yourself. For my own self, I look back on my single days and realize that anything beyond a lengthy kiss was too much for me. Also, remember that guys and girls feel differently about things. A guy may touch a girl's breasts, and she only feels a warm sensation while he is going bananas!

A final word—petting isn't dirty. It may prove to be wrong for you while single. In marriage, petting becomes a very beautiful foreplay, leading up to sex. Yet petting without sex is an empty, frustrating experience. By itself, it doesn't fulfill the need.

### *The Law of Diminishing Returns*

This unsatisfying quality of petting reminds me of what Josh McDowell calls "The law of diminishing returns." That is, each experience leads to other things; holding hands leads to hugging, kissing to caressing, and so on. Where does it stop? Each experience is less fulfilling each time it is repeated. It's a dead-end street without sex. So, why get started down this road?

### *A Bible Passage for Singles*

One of the few Scriptures for singles on sexual behavior is from 1 Thessalonians 4:3–7.

> For this is the will of God, your sanctification; that is, that you abstain from sexual immorality;
> that each of you know how to possess his own vessel in sanctification and honor,
> not in lustful passion, like the Gentiles who do not know God;
> and that no man transgress and defraud his brother in the matter because the Lord is the avenger in all these things, just as we also told you before and solemnly warned you.
> For God has not called us for the purpose of impurity, but in sanctification.

In these challenging verses the apostle Paul gives us some guidelines on the matter of petting and physical involvement. He talks about God's will in verse three. God's will is that we abstain from sexual immorality. Okay, what does that mean? Is a passionate kiss "sexual immorality"? Paul tells us what is proper and what is not by giving the following principles:

1. *Use your body honorably, it is set apart for the Lord* (verse 4).
2. *Don't behave sexually like a pagan. Don't do what everyone else is doing* (verse 5).
3. *Do not transgress your boyfriend/girl friend* (verse 6). To transgress means to go beyond the limits of decency. You'll have to decide what those decent limits are for you. Your heart and conscience will flash the warning when transgression is taking place.
4. *Do not defraud each other* (verse 6). Defrauding is a legal term. (*See* Glossary.) It carries the idea of exciting sexual passions or "turning on" another person sexually. You have "gone too far" when you defraud others or turn them on. Turn ons should be reserved for marriage as foreplay to prepare for intercourse. We can defraud by the clothing we wear, by petting, by

> the movies we see, the books we read, and a hundred other sexually stimulating ways.

The whole point is that God has not "called us for the purpose of impurity, but in sanctification." Save the petting for the pets, and seek to live pure for Him.

# 22 I've Already Lost My Virginity. Can God Forgive?

**I'VE ALREADY LOST MY VIRGINITY. CAN GOD FORGIVE ME? WOULD IT BE HYPOCRITICAL OF ME TO WEAR A WHITE DRESS IN MY WEDDING?**

Learning to live with guilt; that's what too many of us are doing. We walk around in the present with the chains of our past failures and sins hanging heavily around our necks. Nothing destroys today's happiness like yesterday's guilt. The above question addresses itself to the problem of sexual guilt. In one form or another this question has been asked in every dating seminar we've led: "Can I wear a white dress in my wedding?" Wow! I can just feel the heartache in that one!

### *Good News*

Boy, do I have a sunshiny word for your cloudy day! There are some things from our past we have to just live with, but guilt isn't one of them. Jesus Christ our Savior has come to cleanse and heal our guilt—if we allow Him to. However, before we talk about how God heals our guilt and makes us pure again, we need to define some terms like *virginity* and *guilt.*

***Virgins I Have Met***

What is a virgin anyway? The Hebrew word that is used in the Old Testament means "one who lives apart" or "separated." Thus, it meant a woman who was unmarried and lived with her father and mother. A virgin then was a young maiden, unmarried and "undefiled" sexually (*undefiled:* untouched by sin or worldliness). She was an "innocent" maiden. Today we live in a much different kind of world and culture. No longer does the young maiden (say, a sixteen-year-old) stay at home hidden from the wicked world. Today she is out in the world, or the world comes into her home via television and Home Box Office. She may be "undefiled" physically in the sense that she has not had sexual intercourse, but is she "undefiled" in thought or emotions?

Many young men I talk with tell me that some of the "virgins" they have met are pretty "worldly wise." Some girls who haven't gone "all the way" with their bodies have gone all the way in their minds and fantasies. My point is, who is a virgin these days? Far too many of us have seen too much, heard too much, and experienced too much of this sin-saturated society of ours to be innocent.

***Technical Virgins***

Have you lost your virginity? If so, that is a sin, if you lost it to anyone but your wedded mate. Not only is it a sin, it's frequently degrading and shameful. We must not minimize the dignity of purity. When you "lost" your virginity, you did indeed lose something of great value that can never be reclaimed. When it is lost, it is forever lost. In marriage, virginity is not lost; it is exchanged, transformed into the experience of total oneness with your life's partner. However, to sin sexually does not mean you are forever branded "unclean" or impure. We don't stone adulteresses anymore. We forgive them as Jesus did (*see* John 8:1–11). However, to lust in our hearts is to be guilty of sex sin.

Jesus warned us about becoming impure through lust. Any girl or guy who fools around with petting, fondling, and any form of turn ons is only a "technical" virgin. I met one girl who told me she and her boyfriend often lie naked together in bed with much sex play, but she said, "I'm still a virgin. I don't let him go all the way." That's nonsense! She is deceiving herself (him too).

***The Double Standard***

Virginity is not something to be prized by females alone. Young men who are sexually immoral are responsible to God for such behavior. Sexual impurity in young men is not a virtue and a test of manhood. It is sin. What is right for the female is right for the male. Both need God's grace and forgiveness.

***Regaining Innocence***

While it is true that virginity lost can never be reclaimed, that does not mean forgiveness and purity cannot be restored. Jesus said to the woman caught in the very act of adultery, "Go thy way and sin no more" (*see* John 8:11). This is a statement of forgiveness and cleansing. Jesus came to forgive us our sins. This forgiveness includes every kind of sin—even sexual sins. Have you asked Him to forgive you of your sins? If you haven't, do so. Do it now. Put your trust in God's love. Look to the Cross and say, "Lord Jesus, forgive me, cleanse me of my guilt. I trust You now to make me pure in Your sight."

***Seeing What God Sees***

Now, can you believe what you prayed? God says, ". . . Though your sins are as scarlet, they will be as white as snow; Though they are red like crimson, They will be like wool" (Isaiah 1:18). Sins repented of are cleansed. They are removed, blotted out as to become nonexistent. They are forgiven. Forgiven means "sent out of the way." They are no longer an issue between you and God. Therefore, you need to see yourself as God sees you. He sees you as innocent in His sight. Those of us who have committed sex sin need to forgive *ourselves,* because He has forgiven us.

***The Big "A"***

I remember years ago when in high school, we read Hawthorne's *The Scarlet Letter.* I don't know whether today's youth are familiar with this story, but it really relates here. Can a non-virgin wear a white dress without being dishonest? What would be better—to wear a huge scarlet letter *A* across your left breast to advertise your non-virginity? "Adulteress!" How's that for a guilt trip? Wow! I'm sure glad folks don't do that anymore. If they did, I'd go into the Big *A* manufacturing business and sell millions of them every day! No, that's not God's way. What God forgives, He forgets. He receives us gladly. His blood purifies us.

***The White Dress***

What is the point of the traditional white dress anyway? The white dress is a symbol of purity. It is not a symbol of physical virginity. It speaks of the innocence and purity of your love for your husband-to-be. As I see it, any girl who is inwardly pure in heart has every right to wear a wedding gown of *any* color. A lovely girl wrapped up in her gown is a gift she presents to her adoring groom. One final word is needed. You are what you think you are. You can let Satan condemn your heart and fill you with guilt if you choose. (1 John 3:20, 21 says: "in whatever our heart condemns us; for God is greater than our heart, and knows all things. Beloved, if our heart does not condemn us, we have confidence before God.") To do so is to feel worthless, used, and cheap all your days. What is infinitely better is to look to Jesus, receive His love and grace, then walk with your head held high, the past behind you, and a bright future with Him ahead.

# 23 How Do I Apologize to Someone for Past Sexual Sins?

We all know we should make things right with those we've offended or sinned with. This is especially true regarding sexual offenses. One high-school girl told me, "It's really bad when I walk down the hall at school and face my old boyfriend. I'm a Christian now, but when we went together we had sex, and now I can't look him in the eye. I feel so ashamed and guilty." Hey, look, most of us have faced situations similar to that. What we need is some help in knowing how to go to that person and straighten things out, so we can have a clear conscience toward him. Bill Gothard defines a clear conscience as "that inner freedom of spirit toward God and others that comes by knowing that no one can point a finger at you and say, 'You've offended me and you've never asked for my forgiveness.' " The Bible also urges us to have a clear conscience when it says, "Make sure that your conscience is perfectly clear, so that if men speak slanderously of you as rogues they may come to feel ashamed of themselves for abusing you for your good Christian behaviour" (1 Peter 3:16 PHILLIPS).

I suggest some basic steps of action, if you really want to gain a clear conscience. It won't be easy, and the devil himself will hinder you if he can. Only when you are desperate to be rid of guilt will you do something about it. Here's what I told that high-school girl to do:

1. *List and identify the basic offenses.*
   What sins were committed, and what does she need to ask forgiveness for? It helps to write down on paper the things that are bothering you.
2. *Take the offense to God.*
   Clear your conscience with your Heavenly Father. Claim 1 John 1:9 that, "if we confess our sins, he is faithful and righteous to forgive us our sins and to cleanse us from all unrighteousness." Having repented of that sin before God, you are ready for Step 3.
3. *Write out your "speech."*
   To keep you from rambling or "backing out," why don't you write out the wording you'd like to use? It's important not to project blame on the other person by saying, "I let you lead me astray"; or "I let you tempt me"; or, "It was your fault but. . . ." That won't do at all. Simply write down what you should say. Be careful not to be prideful, and don't leave this impression: "Well, I used to be like you, but now I'm better than you." Why not just state the offense, and then say God has convinced you this was wrong and you want to tell him you are sorry and ask for forgiveness. Then ask directly, "Will you forgive me?"
4. *Now you need a method of presentation.*
   Do you now write a letter to that person? Absolutely not! A letter is too impersonal, and it does not demand an answer. Also, a letter documents the sin and can be used for blackmail. The sin you committed was intimate, and it needs to be dealt with intimately. Of course, the best method would be a direct person-to-person, face-to-face confrontation. Set up an appointment or find a convenient place to talk. If this is not possible, the next best thing is a phone call. The conversation need not be long, but can be very direct and to the point. "God has convinced me of how wrong *I* was [not we] in ———. I've called to ask if you will forgive me."

What do you do if the person doesn't forgive you or doesn't see the need to forgive? First, you need to understand why he or she might be unwilling to forgive. It could be their unwillingness is due to a lack of trust. They may question your sincerity. Perhaps they see a lack of real repentance on your part. They want to know if it's for real. Also, their unwillingness may be because your repentance and confession has erased their blame against you, and now he or she is left with the guilt. This often happens. Just know this: you've done what God asked you to do. Your conscience is clear. Whether or not your friend receives your apology is not your responsibility. You can agree with the apostle Paul, "I also do my best to maintain always a blameless conscience both before God and before men" (Acts 24:16).

# 24 Should I Confess to Having Sex Experiences With Other Partners?

**SHOULD A GIRL OR GUY TELL THE PERSON THEY ARE NOW DATING ABOUT PREVIOUS SEXUAL ACTIVITIES WITH OTHER PARTNERS?**

This question is often asked concerning "coming clean" about previous sex sin: "Should I confess it to whomever I may now be dating?" In most cases my answer would be: "No, you should not." I have several good reasons for urging silence rather than confession. Say, for instance, a girl has had an abortion and is now dating several guys. Does she tell *every* guy she dates, "Look, you may not want to continue dating me; I've had an abortion!" Of course not! She might as well wear a scarlet letter *A* on her blouse to announce her wickedness. The problem is *whom* do you tell—which "date" is the right one? Just because you're going steady with someone, does that mean he or she should be told? I suggest a couple of ideas from God's Word about confession that might help.

First, usually, the circle of the offense should determine the circle of the confession. In other words, we seek forgiveness and confess our sin to the persons we've offended. A person who has committed *fornication* (*see* Glossary for definition) with someone should go to *that* person, confess it as sin, and seek forgiveness in order to have a clear conscience toward that person. It is not necessary to go before the church and tell the whole congregation! However, after we have repented of sex sin before God, we definitely should go to the person we sinned against (with) and make it right. Jesus taught us how very important this is. Christ said, "If therefore you are presenting your offering at the altar, and there remember that your brother has something against you, leave your offering there before the altar, and go your way; first be reconciled to your brother, and then come and present your offering" (Matthew 5:23,24). Jesus also taught that if we don't forgive others, God will not forgive us: "And whenever you stand praying, forgive, if you have anything against anyone; so that your Father also who is in heaven may forgive you your transgressions" (Mark 11:25).

Okay, now the question arises, what if you're really serious about someone and planning marriage, etc. Should you tell *that* person about your past before going any further? Of course, situations will vary depending upon the extent of your past promiscuity (*see* Glossary), but normally it is sufficient to say to your girl or boyfriend, "I want to discuss with you some things about my past dating experiences." Then, rather than outline who, where, what, and when, it should be sufficient to say, "I've made some mistakes in my past that God has forgiven, and I've made a whole new start. I'd rather not go into detail, but I wanted you to know I have not been pure sexually. Can you love and accept me as I am?" This approach avoids betraying the confidences of others and still opens up the relationship for discussion, acceptance, and understanding. *Warning:* Should your boy/girl friend insist on details, this reveals an unhealthy attitude on his (her) part. It also reveals an unwillingness to accept you as you are. Now, if there have been some rather severe problems in your past, such as the birth of a child, homosexual acts or desires, or something of that nature, perhaps these areas need to be discussed openly. Openness and honesty are marks of maturity in a love relationship. Such openness can be a test of your friendship. Proverbs says, "He who covers a transgression seeks love, But he who repeats a matter separates intimate friends" (17:9).

# 25 Is There Hope for a Couple That Has "Gone Too Far"?

**IF A COUPLE HAS ALREADY GONE TOO FAR, HOW CAN THEY STRAIGHTEN IT OUT AGAIN? CAN THEY HAVE A GOD-PLEASING RELATIONSHIP?**

"When loves goes wrong, nothin' goes right," the songwriter wrote. That's probably true. One of the saddest questions I am ever asked comes from couples who really care for each other, but their sexual involvement has all but destroyed their courtship. Guilt and confusion hangs over them like a dark cloud. "How can we stop this defrauding and fornicating whenever we're together?"

Well, young friend, it ain't easy! Thomas Wolfe wrote that you can't go home again, and he was right. Innocence lost is not easily recovered. Sexual pleasures are like a man who has never tasted ice cream. When he does taste it, he'll want more the rest of his life. Those who have committed sex sin can testify that stolen apples often taste best. It's difficult to do without it once you've experienced it. This is especially true of those who really love each other.

### *Love Makes It Right*

What often happens is that when two people get involved in sexual impurity, they tend to rationalize that love makes it a noble act of affection. Yet we know in our heart of hearts that this is not true. Saint Augustine said, centuries ago, "It is almost impossible to convince those in love that they are committing fornication." If we can just get past such rationalizing and call sin by its right name, then we can find help.

### *The ABCs of Repentance*

Let me suggest some practical ways to repent of sexual impurity. If a couple really wants to do right, God will help them, whether their impurity is sexual intercourse or petting and fondling. I've put these in *ABCs* to help you remember them.

**A**-*dmit there is a problem.*

Oftentimes a dating couple will suppress the guilt or pretend it isn't there. It seems the girl is more inclined to do this. In her desire to please her boyfriend, she may pretend that sex brings her great joy, when in reality her spirit is being crushed by the shame of it.

Real friendship is characterized by openness and honesty. A couple really in love should be able to admit their problem and discuss it openly.

**B**-*oth must agree that sexual impurity is sin.*

What many times happens is that *both* do not agree about their sexual habits. One thinks it's good; the other doesn't. They become "unequally yoked" (2 Corinthians 6:14 KJV) and much conflict arises. When they are disagreed, they don't communicate, and a wedge begins to be driven between them. Sex, which was meant to be God's gift to end isolation and express intimacy, becomes instead the thing that is destroying their intimacy. The prophet Amos asks, "Can two walk together, except they be agreed?" (3:3 KJV). They must discuss this openly and both agree that what they are doing is against God's Word and God's Law. ". . . the body is not for immorality, but for the Lord . . ." (1 Corinthians 6:13).

**C**-*onsider the reasons you have for dating.*

Couples having sexual problems need to reevaluate their relationship completely. It is sometimes helpful to make a chart of the time spent together in past weeks or months. What do you do together besides "make love"? Do you talk? I mean *really talk* about real things. Do you spend creative time together? Does your time together bless you and others around you? Are you better together than you are apart? Is your friendship positive or negative? Some couples will have to admit that sex is their *main* reason for being together. This is a destructive friendship and needs to be reconstructed.

**D**-*ate with planning and purpose.*

A couple can reevaluate *where* they spend time together. Giving careful attention and planning to where you will go and what you will do can avoid many traps which encourage excessive petting.

**E**-*arnestly pray about it together.*

Spiritual problems need spiritual resources. When you fail God sexually, repent of it (together) and seek His cleansing. Pray about it daily, regularly, until God's grace is sufficient.

**F**-*ailure to resolve the problem must result in decision to break up.*

A wise person once said, "Better tears than scars." If you can't honor God with your bodies, then better to dissolve the relationship than to forfeit fellowship with your Heavenly Father.

This matter of breaking up will be discussed in the next chapter.

# 26 How Can You Break Up and Still Be Friends When You've Had Sex Together?

Breaking up is hard to do. It was when I was young, and it still is today. We don't like to hurt people we care about; but sometimes a dating relationship just doesn't work out for a number of reasons and it's time to call it quits.

Breaking up is even harder when you've said words like *I love you,* or when you've made a sexual commitment. Both love and sex are words and deeds which speak of lasting "forever"-type commitments. Then, to have to retract them and admit you were wrong or mistaken can really be tough. How do you break up "gracefully"? Can two people break up and still be friends?

Yes, I think you can. Especially if the two of you are really friends. In fact, breaking up the courtship may be the only way to prove (or disprove) the depth of the friendship. Often a girl fears breaking off a sexual relationship for fear of losing her guy. If so, she's using her body as bait to keep her guy. Tragically, if sex is what's keeping him, he's not worth having. At least, the relationship is not worth saving.

As mentioned previously, Thomas Carlyle said a long time ago, "True friends, like ivy and the wall, stand together or fall together." Changing the type of relationship you now have to one God wants you to have will let you know how true the friendship really is.

*Breaking up* is a phrase I held suspect for many years. Why do we call it that? Probably because among the immature the separation or closing of a dating relationship is a violent, angry, emotional parting, in which people are hurt and there is very little understanding of feelings. *Breaking up* describes a selfish, shallow kind of relationship in which there was little real communication. Friends shouldn't break up. They should come to a mutual understanding.

### *Hurt, Yes; Anger, No*

This does not mean someone doesn't feel genuine hurt or pain of loss. When two people break off what has been a serious courtship, it often leaves a deep wound. The healing help of the Great Physician can make the healing time more bearable. Yes, you can bear the hurt and loss. You may weep, but God will store up your tears in a bottle (Psalms 56:8) so precious are they to Him. However, anger and bitterness tell me two people have not talked out the reasons and come to an understanding of "I want what's best for both of us."

How can you break off a courtship that needs to end? Here are some suggestions.

### *The Direct Approach*

Breaking up is easier if both of you agree. It is much more difficult if only *you* are convinced. At any rate, tell your girl/boyfriend how you feel, face-to-face. Do so in a neutral place, without the romantic "trappings." See if you can openly discuss it without anger. Try to pray about it together, if possible. Remember this: the decision to end the relationship must be made *before* you discuss it. As John White says in *Eros Defiled,* "The only discussion has to do not with *whether* or even with *when,* but with *how.*"

### *The Indirect Approach*

If there have not been serious problems between you (such as fornication or defrauding), breaking up may be done indirectly by just tapering off the time together. Without hurting feelings, just suggest you not see so much of each other. Make yourself unavailable for a dating relationship. Sometimes this is enough to cool off a situation where one person is getting too serious.

### *Involve Others*

If the situation calls for it, you might consider bringing in a third person for support and objectivity. If you are a teenager, you could involve a parent, a schoolteacher, your youth minister, or even a friend. Sometimes it is helpful to bring in an adult if you are a teenager and an ex-boyfriend (girl friend) just won't leave you alone and keeps hanging on.

One last word here—if sexual sins are a part of your dating past, you can be sure God wants that to change. Don't hang on out of "obligation" because you've had sex. Better to confess the sin than to compound the sin out of some foolish sense of duty. Your duty is to God first.

# 27 If a Couple Has Had Sex, Will Getting Married Make It Right?

**MY GIRL FRIEND AND I BEGAN DATING ABOUT TWO YEARS AGO WHEN WE WERE IN HIGH SCHOOL. ONE THING LED TO ANOTHER AND FINALLY WE WENT ALL THE WAY. WE ARE BOTH CHRISTIANS AND WE LOVE EACH OTHER, BUT WE BOTH FEEL VERY GUILTY ABOUT HAVING SEX. IF WE GO AHEAD AND GET MARRIED, WILL THAT MAKE IT RIGHT?**

No, it will not. Now don't panic; let me explain my bluntness. Getting married cannot forgive a sin or right a wrong relationship or deed. But then no human effort can forgive a single sin or undo a wrong deed. Only the Lord Jesus can "make things right." That is done through confession and repentance of sin. That's better and less expensive than getting married!

### *Sources or Symptoms*

Getting married may be what this couple needs to do. Remember, Saint Paul said, "Better to marry than burn with passion." Marriage does many wonderful things for people but forgiving sin isn't one of them. A couple that is having sex whether they are in love, engaged, or whatever, will not get rid of guilt through a wedding ring. Getting married doesn't touch the symptoms. Tim Stafford, in discussing sex among engaged couples, makes this statement:

> Let's take the ultimate case. Suppose I were getting married June 29, and I and my fiancée got carried away the night before, June 28. Would I be in the wrong just because I was a few hours ahead of the scheduled ceremony? I doubt this kind of premarital sex poses a serious threat to marriage, and therefore I doubt if God is most concerned about it. But there is a principle involved—cheating a nickel on your income tax is still cheating . . . for violating promises we made to God or each other, my fiancée and I would need to be forgiven.
>
> *A Love Story* (Zondervan)

Notice this statement—they need to be forgiven. Marriage is not the cure-all for sex sin; repentance is.

***Marry for the Right Reasons***

My point here is that it is not right to marry just to legalize sex. That's the old "caught in the act," shotgun-wedding scene. It reminds me of the old movie where the pretty blonde farmer's daughter comes climbing down out of the hayloft with straw in her hair saying to her beau, "Well, you just have to marry me now." That kind of thinking wasn't good then and it stinks now. I doubt that God appreciates such a degrading view of marriage. People should marry because they feel they belong together in spirit, soul, and body.

***A Final Word***

I'd like to add another thought here. Many couples feel guilt about sex sin, as indeed they will if the Holy Spirit is allowed to touch their hearts. One of the reasons they feel this way is because to *most* girls, sex is an expression of a love commitment. A college survey was taken of several thousand students who were experienced sexually. They were asked to list their reasons for having sex. Ninety-five percent of the young men said they had sex for either pleasure or curiosity. Only 5 percent of the males said they had sex to show real love commitment. However, the statistics were reversed among the non-virgin coeds interviewed. Ninety-five percent of the girls said they had sex with their guy because they loved him; only 5 percent said sex was merely physical pleasure or curiosity. How about that! What does that tell you? It tells me that women need love and commitment, and that sex is not a plaything with the female gender. Fellows, we can put our gal under a tremendous guilt trip with our loose attitudes toward her body. He who plays loose with sex is playing to lose with sex.

# 28 Should I Stop Dating a Non-Virgin?

**AN UNUSUAL THING HAS HAPPENED TO ME. I AM A COLLEGE JUNIOR AND I'VE BEEN DATING THIS WONDERFUL CHRISTIAN GIRL FOR SEVERAL MONTHS. WE'VE GROWN VERY CLOSE, AND ONLY THIS WEEK SHE TOLD ME THAT SHE WAS NOT A VIRGIN AND HAD EVEN HAD AN ABORTION. I AM PLANNING TO ENTER THE MINISTRY AFTER SEMINARY AND SHE THINKS WE SHOULD COOL IT BECAUSE OF HER PAST SINS. I REALLY CARE FOR HER AND WANT TO CONTINUE TO DATE HER. IS SHE RIGHT? SHOULD WE STOP DATING? IS THERE NO FUTURE FOR US?**

A young preacher boy falling in love with a wonderful girl with a "past." Tough decision. I'm hard put to offer sound wisdom. Should we forgive and forget, or is she right—will her past catch up with them years later? It does happen, you know. Your past sins can come out of the closet to haunt you like ghosts. Should this young man marry this girl, they together have the reputation of Christ to uphold. Would her past sin be a taint on his ministry if it became public?

### *Go, and Sin No More*

Of course, God has forgiven her, and it seems she has grown from her mistakes and wants to please God in the future. It speaks well for her that she has the character to admit her feelings and doesn't want to hurt him. Perhaps what he should do is what God has done—forgive her just as Jesus forgave the woman caught in adultery (John 8:1–11). Certainly they cannot be real friends without this forgiveness. He must not only *forgive,* but he must *forget* it as well. Forgiveness means the deed is no longer an issue between you. It's a dead issue. *That's* forgiveness, when it includes remembering it no more. My own feeling is that if they indeed continue dating and God leads them along the way, that her past need not be a hindrance to their future happiness and successful ministry together. In fact, her past can build character in her that God can use in years ahead. Those who have been hurt the most and healed the best often become the greatest healers and helpers.

### *Is the Problem Resolved?*

The young man who wrote this note didn't tell me if he and this "wonderful Christian girl" were having sexual problems together. Maybe she is telling him about her past sexual activity as a warning. She may be afraid she cannot handle another romantic involvement. Her confession could be her way of voicing her fears of her weakness. It is possible that she could pull the two of them down spiritually because of her temptation. I don't know that this is true, but it has happened before. Her warning—if it is a warning—could be her way of saying, "Help me, I don't want to be hurt again, and I don't want to hurt you or our friendship."

### *Set the Boundaries*

This brings me to a good word for all of us. As any friendship grows in dating, two people discover things about each other. Sometimes they are secret things about kinks in our armor. A girl may discover her fellow is subject to sexual temptation very easily or vice versa. The issue isn't "Should I date a non-virgin?" but rather, "Can I help my friend become more like Jesus?" If a couple talks about their sexual needs, weaknesses, and so on, they can then set some goals and boundaries to help them avoid falling into the same habits and pitfalls.

For example, a young person who has had sexual intercourse and been very intimate with a lover may have to go through "withdrawal" for a long time. In petting, he or she must "know thyself"; that is, know what turns you on to the point of no return. A couple should help each other by avoiding situations and activities that are a trap. We've discussed this earlier, but the non-virgin has a tougher row to hoe than the "innocent" youth.

There may need to be some reconditioning to discover other ways of showing affection and love without a great deal of sexual contact. It can be done, and God will help you and bless you for trying.

# 29 Is It All Right to Use Contraceptives?

**IS IT ALL RIGHT TO USE CONTRACEPTIVES TO PREVENT PREGNANCY? CAN SINGLE GIRLS GO ON THE PILL TO PLAY IT SAFE? SHOULD PARENTS ENCOURAGE THEIR DAUGHTERS TO DO SO?**

The use of contraceptives to prevent pregnancy is a loaded issue, and you'll find many differing views even among committed Christians. However, before I share my own thoughts, it has occurred to me that some of my younger readers may not understand fully what contraceptives are all about. So I will first explain them and then talk about their use among single people. This liberated generation on the Pill needs some guidance from God's Word on this matter. The Pill is not paradise. It does not and has not solved our sexual fears of unwanted pregnancies. Nearly ½ million teenage abortions each year testify to that fact.

### *Contraceptives—Take Your Pick*

Dr. Ed Wheat and his wife, Gaye, have written a very fine sex manual for Christians, *Intended for Pleasure* (Revell), in which they discuss fully the use of contraceptives. I recommend the book to engaged couples. Dr. & Mrs. Wheat recommended three considerations in choosing a method of contraception: *safety, ef-*

*fectiveness,* and *your own personal taste.* Of course, there are those who are opposed to any use of contraceptives. Roman Catholic theology has debated this heavily in recent years. For my part, it's a dead issue. Millions of Catholics disagree with the papal edicts and are using contraceptives for planned parenthood. In our crowded world, I feel Christians have a moral imperative to limit the size of their families. Also, we are to provide for what we beget, which encourages limited childbirth. If you agree with this, what types of contraceptives are available?

***The Miracle Pill***

The oral contraceptive otherwise known as the "Pill" has set women "free" all over the world. The problem with the Pill is that thousands of teenage girls have gotten on it without medical counsel and failed to take it properly. One sixteen-year-old girl told me, "I don't know how I got pregnant. I took my Pill every time *right after* my boyfriend and I had sex!" Wow, what a dummy! Yet, thousands of kids imitate her. The Pill isn't a candy miracle cure for sexual promiscuity. Any oral contraceptive requires disciplined, regulated usage, recommended by a physician.

Dr. Wheat explains:

> The oral-contraceptive method calls for a woman to take a contraceptive pill or tablet every day for twenty-one days. A woman beginning to use this method takes the first pill five days after the start of her menstrual period. She then takes one pill every day until she takes twenty-one pills. Then she stops taking the pills, and within two or three days her period should begin. Seven days after taking the last tablet, she begins taking the pill again for twenty-one days and repeats the cycle. This routine continues month after month for as long as the woman wishes to prevent pregnancy.

Other less popular forms of contraception include the *vaginal diaphragm with spermicides, vaginal spermicides without dia-*

*phragm, the intrauterine device* (IUD), or the rhythm method. Married couples must consult a physician and determine what is safest, most effective and pleasurable for them. But what about birth control among single people?

### *An Ounce of Prevention*

Numerous high-school girls have told me their mother took them to the doctor and put them on birth control, usually the Pill. Many of these girls come from Christian families, whose parents are leaders in the church. One such mother told me, "Look, preacher, an ounce of prevention is worth a pound of cure. I don't want my daughter coming up pregnant. The Pill sure beats an abortion." Well, she is right. The Pill does beat an abortion by nine miles. However, that's like giving poison to a child to prevent cancer. He gets clobbered either way! The solution to unwanted pregnancy is virginity or abstinence, not arming the youth of America with the Pill and condoms! May God have mercy on parents like that! For my part, providing birth control for your children is an endorsement of their sin. It's saying, "If you are going to do it, just don't get caught." Listen, friends, the evil of fornication is not in the "getting caught." It's in the irresponsibility of the act and the misuse of the body. God isn't fooled, deceived, or appeased, because we use birth control during our fornication.

What is needed is a responsible, mature, even godly attitude toward our bodies and each other. Birth control within marriage can be a blessing that frees a couple to enjoy sex without fear of unwanted pregnancy. However, birth control for singles is just not a solution to the real problem. It's only a remedy that deals with symptoms rather than causes.

It may be recommended by clinics and governmental agencies for wayward youth, but it is not the answer for those who want to please God. Birth control must not be an excuse to sin or to make sin easier.

*ABORTION—*

*Legal, illegal, open or secret,*
*privately funded or federally funded,*
*however you want to describe it—*
*it is a tragedy.*
*Someone made a mistake and acted irresponsibly*
*with dynamic life-forces.*

# 30 My Girl Friend Is Pregnant. What Should We Do?

**I'VE BEEN DATING THIS GIRL FOR A LONG TIME AND WE PLANNED TO GET MARRIED SEVERAL YEARS FROM NOW, BUT I'M ONLY SEVENTEEN AND HAVE TWO MORE YEARS OF HIGH SCHOOL. ANYWAY, WE JUST FOUND OUT SHE'S PREGNANT. WE HAVEN'T TOLD ANYBODY YET. SHOULD WE GO AHEAD AND GET MARRIED NOW? WHAT ARE OUR OPTIONS?**

A few years ago an attractive young couple came to my office. The young man, a junior in high school, told me his story. He made the above statement that he and the pretty teenager sitting beside him were "in trouble." What should they do? Situations like this put gray hairs on my head prematurely, but, thank God, I'd counseled situations like this before. As we talked, I tried to explain to these two the painful and difficult options that were theirs. How pitiful! Two kids who have never made a major decision in their young lives, now faced with these all-important, life-changing decisions.

### *To Marry or Not to Marry*

The young man suggested he do the honorable thing and marry the girl. Remarkably, *she* was opposed to that suggestion. She said, "I'm so confused. Johnny, I'm not even sure I want to get married. At least not now, and not for that reason. I want you to marry me because you *want* to, not because it's your duty or because you feel you *have* to." I was now feeling better about this whole thing. This girl had some smarts about her. She at least knew marriage was more than legalized fornication! No couple should marry just to give the poor little baby a name. Society will name the baby through an adoption agency. Marriage is often the worst solution—especially when the couple is so young and immature. Making it "right" doesn't always mean to marry. Making it *right* may mean honest confession of sin, repentance, breaking up, and seeking other options which we will discuss.

### *A Family Affair*

I asked these kids when they were going to tell their parents about the pregnancy. Of course, they were scared and dreaded facing their parents. "Would you like me to set up a meeting and be there to tell your parents for you?" I asked. Very relieved, they agreed. Of course the parents had to be told, and *now*—not weeks later. You see, many young people who fool around with sex never think of the broad implications of their behavior. What they do alone in the dark affects many other people. Their private affair is in reality a family affair. What they do together sexually is never just for the two of them. Sex carries with it social responsibility. Frequently couples in that mad moment of passion are blinded to the real world. They feel only the thrill of the moment—that is, until they are faced with the realities that now faced this couple. Well, we did meet with both parents together that very day and their private affair became a very sad family affair.

### *What Now? Punt?*

The conversation was painful but necessary. Both sets of parents agreed that marriage was not the answer. However, I've seen it go the other way too. I've seen the girl's father outraged that his little girl has been defiled (forgetting that it takes two to tango) and want to strangle the boy. I've seen parents *demand* a wedding to save face (usually theirs, not the kids). It's amazing, but a crisis like this either brings out the best or the worst in people. It's been said, "A crisis does not make a friendship; it only reveals it." How very true. Even members of families can become very unfriendly over sex sin. Okay, marriage was not the solution for these two kids, who really were not ready for that kind of commitment. What do we do next? Punt? We almost did. Both mothers were in favor of an abortion for the girl. (That's punting with a capital *P*.)

### *Stay Cool, Counselor*

It's at this point that I need all the help I can get to stay cool. God in His heaven knows my violent reaction to abortion for convenience sake. In 1979 over 300,000 teenage girls had abortions! Over a million abortions were performed in America in 1979. Not a fraction of these was to protect the health of the mother. Most were performed to free the mother of the responsibility of motherhood. (Statistics have been increasing every year for the last five years, as abortion laws have become increasingly more lenient.) This book is not the place for me to get on my soapbox and air *all* my views about abortion. Others have already done so and in a manner far superior to what I could do. I have listed suggested reading under "Abortion" in the Glossary at the back of this book. Nevertheless, I'll tell you what I told this girl and the parents. Abortion as a means to dodge the embarrassment and shame of an untimely or unwanted pregnancy by two irresponsible teenagers is not only unjustified, it is a sin. It ought to be a crime. Abortions of this type may be legal or illegal, depending upon the laws of your state. In some states and countries like Japan, Canada, and various European countries, abortions can be performed by qualified medical staff. All that is needed is a request (demand) by the pregnant female. She can walk into an abortion clinic, be examined, scheduled for a simple removal of the pregnancy (if aborted early), and after a few hours, walk out—as easy as a trip to the dentist. Perhaps that's a part of the problem: it's all *too* convenient, *too* easy. We're hearing too much these days about freedom and not enough about reponsibility. All those in favor of "abortion upon demand" talk incessantly about the mother's rights and freedom, yet very few are talking about the rights and freedom of the unborn child.

Most Christians object to abortion upon demand of the mother. Many are not happy about abortion for any cause, regardless if it's carried out by capable physicians for medical or psychiatric reasons.

### *Therapeutic Abortions*

Some feel there may be grounds for abortion when the life or health (mental or physical) of the mother is at stake. Some situations such as rape, incest, or the use of damaging drugs by the mother that would cause deformity in the fetus are cited as examples. However, an abortion for the reasons these parents in this chapter discussion were contemplating would be counterproductive. For this girl to have an abortion would do more than destroy a potential life—she would be destroying her integrity and that of her parents. To the surprise of both mothers this girl again surprised us by her integrity. She flatly refused to consider an abortion as an option. As her mother wept and felt sorry for herself, this teenage girl let it be known she wanted to carry this child through to childbirth. Remarkable! I never cease to be amazed at the courage of young people! *God bless them!*

### *Tarnished but Not Broken*

Her reaction leads me to say again that those who have committed sex sin and been caught at it (by pregnancy) are not necessarily evil people. I am not justifying fornication or adultery but want to illustrate the fact that many others are just as guilty or more so. Thousands of girls are walking around carrying the guilt of their sexual promiscuity or the guilt of an abortion. Perhaps nobody knows about it, but the truth is they lacked the courage to face their failure as this young lady did. She was unwilling to compound her sin by adding abortion to the list. I salute her and may her tribe increase. She was tarnished but not broken.

### *Who Wants This Baby?*

All right, if you don't terminate the pregnancy, then you let it continue. What then do we do about the baby? This brings up the options three and four. These are always the most difficult to accept, but are perhaps the most noble and rewarding in the long run. After much discussion, it became obvious that this girl's feelings toward her baby ran much deeper than her feelings for her boyfriend. She was not sure she loved him (in a mature love that included marriage) but she knew she would and could love this baby. Yet, truthfully, if she kept this baby as an eighteen-year-old girl, her problems were going to be very real. We talked frankly about these problems. She was unmarried, her education was incomplete, and she would have to live with her parents. She would have to raise her child *against* the wishes of her parents. She would be cut off from her school friends and school life. All of which is a tremendous amount of pressure to put on a young girl. Motherhood has its own set of pressures without all of that added to it.

### *A Compromise That Didn't Work*

Parents can be right; they are also capable of being selfish and very wrong. In this case they misjudged their daughter. Listening to her parents' pleadings, this girl settled upon a compromise. She agreed to carry the baby and then give it away to an adoption agency. She would give birth to this child, but never see it, hold it, or love it. This she did, but not without tragic emotional results. In the years that followed, this very conscientious girl tried to commit suicide several times. She has been crushed by the reality that she "abandoned" her baby to strangers. It is now very clear that she and her parents made a mistake. The compromise hasn't worked. *Don't misunderstand me here.* In some cases, the right decision is to do as she did. Many girls have given their babies away to agencies. The agencies in turn put the children into families that have been carefully picked out. Most of these girls carry on with their lives and learn from this experience. Some, like this girl, just cannot cope with it.

### *To Have and Hold*

She would have been better off to have kept her baby, regardless of the problems. Knowing her strong spirit, she would have handled it. I know another girl who did keep the baby. At the time of her pregnancy, she was about twenty-two years old. She came to me for counsel. She shared with me that she hardly knew the father. It was only a passing sexual encounter. She decided to have the baby and keep it. And she did. I'll never forget the way she dealt with her "disgrace." She told her parents, asked their forgiveness, then began her public life as an unwed mother. Those who knew her were touched by her contrite heart and her repentant spirit. She was ashamed of her sin and had learned her lesson the hard way. It changed her life. Yet, she was not ashamed of the child she carried. She believed that her baby was God's gift to her. It was God's heavenly sandpaper to polish and perfect her character. The day her baby was born, I was there to greet her when she came to her room. I'll never forget the joy on her face as she held her baby boy. Wow! It was beautiful. She had turned adversity into triumph. She married a fine Christian man a year or so later, and God has blessed their marriage. That daddy loves that boy!

### *The Best Solution*

I wish I could say I always know the best solution to unwanted pregnancies (among unmarried people). I don't know what's best. I just know what's worst! When a girl finds herself in that situation she needs wise, unbiased, *biblical* counsel. Even then she'll have to make her own decision and live with it the rest of her life. An ounce of prevention is always worth a pound of cure!

## *A LETTER TO ANN LANDERS*

Dear Ann Landers:

I am only 17 and I have succeeded in messing up my life completely. Ted and I went steady for six months and we were sure we were in love. One thing led to another. We promised each other dozens of times "Never again"—but we just couldn't stay away from each other. You know how it is with teen-agers—once they start getting very, very intimate it is almost impossible to stop, especially if they keep seeing each other and think they are in love. But now you can probably guess the rest. I became pregnant. Ted and I both quit school and got married right away. Our friends dropped us like hot coals.

My folks don't want anything to do with me now. They say I have disgraced the family. I guess they are right. They also say they warned me about going steady and seeing so much of Ted. They are right about THAT, too. Ted's folks feel pretty much the same as my folks and I can't blame them. I see no hope for the future. The baby cries all the time and I am a nervous wreck. I feel sorry for the baby because I am a poor mother. I guess I'm just too young for all this. We live in a terrible place. It is damp and dingy and rundown, but it's the best we can afford. Ted never says anything but I know he must hate me, because he feels I got him into this. He always wanted to go to college and amount to something. Of course now he never will.

There are times when I think this is all a bad dream, and I will wake up in my parents' nice home, and go to school with the kids I like so much. But I know too well that those days are over for me and I am stuck. I am not writing for advice, Ann, it is too late for that. I am just writing in the hope that you will print my letter for the benefit of other teen-agers who think they know it all—like I did.

# 31 Why Do So Many Teenage Marriages Not Work Out?

Depending upon whose statistics you read, it is estimated that three out of four teenage marriages will end in divorce *before* the couple move into their twenties. Teenage marriages just seem to be doomed to fail. Why?

In *Intended for Pleasure,* Dr. Wheat gives the following reasons for teen marriage failure:

> First, because teenagers in most cases cannot separate from their parents and become independent. Second, teenagers have changing value systems, and they do not yet know what they will want in a mate. Qualities later surface which were not apparent when the young people married. This is because character develops as a response to responsibility or adversity. There is no way of predicting with accuracy how a teenager will respond to the difficulties and demands of married life in the years ahead.

It's obvious from reading the above brief paragraph that this Christian counselor and medical doctor isn't too high on teenage marriage. He has some valid points. *Most* teenagers are not mature enough for a marriage commitment. Marriage carries with it profound responsibilities, which even mature adults struggle with.

My main objection to young people rushing into marriage centers around this area of personality development. Growing up, learning responsibility, self-acceptance, and self-confidence takes time. Too often young people become emotionally attached to each other and even emotionally dependent ("I can't live without her [him]!") on each other *before* they've had a chance to "go it alone." Each of us needs to learn the answers to such questions as, "Who am I?"; "What can I do?"; and "Why am I here?" before we start changing *our* children's diapers!

Marriage is a joining of two into one soul and flesh. Marriage makes bad arithmetic—one plus one equals one! Therefore, when two teenagers join together, they need to have had time to develop each individual "one" before they merge into a new "oneness." If two undeveloped self-hoods marry, what you get is a half-baked whole! That's what Dr. Wheat was saying. We need to learn "aloneness" before we commit ourselves to "togetherness."

If that isn't enough reason to discourage teenage marriage, let me go a step further. In addition to the psychological problems, there are the obvious financial and social difficulties. How does the teenage husband support his wife? He does so one of three ways. He may move in with his or her parents, which is a bummer from the start. Jesus said in marriage a man *leaves* his father and mother and joins his wife. He did not say he brings his wife to move in with them! Their second alternative is to quit school to support the two of them. There are then all kinds of social difficulties which follow. Being "cut off" from one's peers can be very hard to take for many teenagers. Even if they do continue in school, being married makes them "different" from the rest of the gang. A third solution is for the couple's parents to support them. This too is no good. A couple gets married to be *separate* from parents. Marriage is an adult act of independence, the forming of a new family. When a teenage couple is financially and emotionally dependent on parents, they will usually find that there are strings attached to such help. Parents still tend to treat them as dependents (which they are).

Modern society is making it harder and harder for young marrieds to get by financially. The job market is highly competitive. A teenage couple thinking of marriage should take the *long* look, not just the *short* look. They should ask themselves some realistic questions: "Should we wait till we've finished [or furthered] our education?" "Will we be able to live on the social scale we're used to, or will early marriage hinder that?" "Are we ready for the daily pressures marriage brings?" "Can we do for ourselves what others have been doing for us?" These and other questions are more important than a couple's hot blood, or young love that drives them to be together. Remember, God's Word says, "Love is *patient*..." (1 Corinthians 13:4 italics mine).

One other word—Christian teenagers must take seriously God's Word to children. He says, "Honor thy father and thy mother." Good advice. Whatever your plans regarding love, courtship, and marriage, such plans are a family affair. You do not just marry *each other*—you marry each other's *tribe!* You marry into *families.* Parents must be consulted and included. That is God's command to us.

# 32 What Does the Bible Teach About Exotic Sexual Activities, Even After Marriage?

Without exception, the question about oral sex (*see* Glossary) is asked wherever we go. In seminars in every part of the country, regardless of the age group, young people in junior-high school as well as in college want to know if oral sex is a normal sexual activity for a Christian. Some even want to know if oral sex is acceptable among single people as a substitute for sexual intercourse.

In reply to such questions, we'd better determine what is meant by "normal" sex. The Christian who wishes to please the Father above should beware of seeking what is so-called normal by the world's standards in anything. Because *normal* only describes "the way things are"; it says nothing about the way things *should* be. In other words, normal sex may not be sex as God intended it. Normal sex may not be good sex—only kinky.

In speaking to this very subject of oral sex, leading Christian psychologist John White says, "Today in our feverish pursuit of sensual pleasure we are rediscovering a broad range of erotic pleasures which have flourished as each civilization has entered into its phase of decadence. Christian couples are enjoying such delights as oro-genital sex. . . . Is such sex normal?"

Some Christian writers would reply with a simple *yes.* They would say that among married couples, anything they do together sexually is sacred. This position is stated in Dr. and Mrs. Ed Wheat's book *Intended for Pleasure.* I've given much thought to this idea and have finally rejected it.

Such an answer is too simplistic. Scripture teaches us that the purpose of marriage and sex is to end isolation: "It is not good for the man to be alone . . ." (Genesis 2:18). Sex is a means of communion and oneness. Sex can break down the barriers that exist between two people—or it can erect barriers. It all depends upon the attitude you bring to it. Erotic sexual pleasure is the most superficial benefit of sex. It brings only the joy of the moment. Therefore, oral sex, to be beneficial, must not be a thing sought as an end in itself. As a part of the foreplay and arousal that leads to the marital bliss of sexual intercourse, such activities are acceptable *if* both partners find pleasure in them. When a husband and wife engage in any sexual activity that is for their mutual joy and is a part of the process whereby they learn communion and spiritual oneness, that activity fulfills God's purpose for sex.

However, this does not mean that "anything goes." The God-ordained expression of sexual climax is sexual intercourse.

The penis was designed to accommodate the vagina—not other body cavities (openings). Also, procreation may be a secondary purpose for sex, but it is a *God*-ordained purpose and should not be discarded in favor of kinky sex.

In conclusion, what I am saying is that there is no simple answer to this question. What we need to see is that any form of oro-genital sex which is not a part of an ongoing interpersonal sexual relationship, and which does not lead to sexual intercourse between a husband and wife, is "abnormal" in the Christian sense.

# LOVE

*The more one loves,*
*The better we are, and*
*The greater our friendships are,*
*The dearer we are to God.*

*Jeremy Taylor*

# 33 What Is the Difference Between Infatuation and Real Love?

A fourteen-year-old talked to me after a session on dating just last week. In tearful terms she told me how her heart was breaking because a ninth-grade boy she was "in love with" had broken up with her. Expressing her agony, she said, "I'm just going to die if I can't get him back."

I doubt it! I did tell her that, and that she will get over this one and a few more before lasting, real love comes along. She is infatuated with this ninth-grade superstar, not in love with him. There is a difference. Of course, infatuation is real, and oftentimes as strong an emotion as love. Puppy love feels exactly like the real thing. It is especially real to the puppy who's got a bad case of it. It can make the puppy act like a sick dog! There's no experience quite like a seventh-grade boy "in love" with the pretty little blonde sitting in front of him in English class. He can't eat, sleep; he walks around in a trance; he stares at her soft curls, and longs to touch her—but dares not. That kid is lovesick. But it isn't real love; he's infatuated—and he'll get over it, like getting over a bad cold. Perhaps you've had this sickness recently, or maybe you've got it now. What is needed is a good diagnosis, examination, and recommended treatment. You really do need to get cured of infatuation, so that you can move on to a healthier way of life—real love.

### *Infatuation Diagnosed*

Infatuation is not confined to the very young. Adults catch it also. Not as often, but some do. What is infatuation? What's the difference between infatuation and genuine love?

First of all, infatuation is an emotion. It is a shallow emotional feeling. It is love of emotion. "She makes me feel good." "When he looks at me, I just get chills all over my body." Such are the vibes of infatuation. Real love is deeper than emotion. Real love involves the will. Real love continues when the feelings are gone and the vibes aren't there. Infatuation is just *love of emotion;* real love is *devotion.*

Second, infatuation is something you "fall into." Webster's defines *infatuation* as "being carried away by unreasoning passion or attraction." It sounds like something you'd "fall in," like a trap! When I hear of "love at first sight," I think of a guy seeing the girl, and she pounces on him and zaps him with her magic love potion. He's now "got it." He's "fallen" in love. No. He's *infatuated.* It's a madness based on "unreasoning passion or attraction." Real love is a growing experience, based on mutually shared interests, beliefs, attitudes, and goals. You can be infatuated with someone you don't even know (a movie star), and have never met. It is based on physical attraction or popularity. Love isn't like that at all. I'm not saying physical attraction is bad. Infatuation *can* lead to love, but it isn't love. Too many times we call infatuation *love.* Love is a very precious gem and not to be merchandised with all the costume junk sold in discount stores. Don't call your "unreasoning passion" love—call it *infatuation.*

### *Give and Take*

Third, infatuation, though often called love, is really the opposite of real love. Infatuation is a selfish emotion. Infatuation is "in love with love" rather than in love *with another person.* Real love is giving, not taking. Love is more selfless than selfish. Infatuation is possessive. It translates as *I want you* rather than *I love you.* When we are infatuated, we want our love to "belong" to us; we are jealous of anyone who threatens our possession. We want our beloved to belong to us even if he or she doesn't want to. Our girl/boyfriend is for our pleasure, whether they like it or not! Of course, this isn't love at all. I see this in lads "going steady" during the early teen years. Going steady is kind of "protection of private property." It's usually infatuation, and it's insecure and selfish.

Fourth, infatuation doesn't last. It is temporary. It will pass with time and changing circumstances. It is weakened by time and separation. True love is strengthened by separation. It is what Tim Stafford calls *forever love.* He says in *A Love Story:* "It's the kind of love that lasts forever, because it's love that refuses to be stopped by hurt feelings, by failures, or by attraction you feel for a third person. Forever love doesn't just happen to you. It's something you decide on, and commit yourself to."

Okay, enough of what love isn't. We've diagnosed the sickness of infatuation, now to prescribe the cure. What is the genuine article? What are the marks of this *forever love?*

### *Before I Say, "I Love You"*

If you listen to much rock music you know about "love" songs. There would be no music today were there no more love songs. Love is in the air (waves). Yet, if you listen closely you'll discover most of what they are singing about is not "forever" love. It's something less than that. Not all we call love is really love. What I want to suggest is that you save that word for the real thing. Love is more than sexual excitement or infatuation. I agree with the words of John White in *Eros Defiled* when he says of love:

> Love is the fulfilling of the law. It truly sums up biblical morality. But the love that fulfills the law is not the glazed, heavy-breathed stirring in the groins that clouds your judgment and seduces your will as you copulate. It is not the love that you *make*.... Love is more than pity, greater than compassion,

> deeper than understanding and more positive than self-denial. It is the agape love of 1 Corinthians 13, the love that originates in the heart of God. The love that cannot stop when the love object ceases to please.

What we need to do is put this "forever," God-kind of love under the microscope and look it over. When we understand it, we can seek it, work toward it, and commit ourselves to it. The marks of real love are described in First Corinthians 13, verses 4–7. Here it is from The Living Bible—the "in spite of" kind of love:

> Love is very patient and kind, never jealous or envious, never boastful or proud, never haughty or selfish or rude. Love does not demand its own way. It is not irritable or touchy. It does not hold grudges and will hardly even notice when others do it wrong. It is never glad about injustice, but rejoices whenever truth wins out. If you love someone you will be loyal to him no matter what the cost. You will always believe in him, always expect the best of him, and always stand your ground in defending him.
>
> PAUL THE APOSTLE

What a remarkable paragraph. I'm glad God said all that! Our Heavenly Father Himself has described His very own nature to us, for God *is* love! Let's take a look at these characteristics of love and before you say, "I love you" again, compare your commitment to the real thing. (Obviously, wherever I've written "him" also refers to "her" in these paragraphs.)

### *Love Is Very Patient*

When you love someone, you have enough maturity to accept him as he is. It's not the *potential* person you love, but the *actual* person; mistakes, flaws, and all.

***Love Is Kind***

It is constructive, positive, and uplifting. Love sees needs and seeks ways to help improve the other's life. It is not negative and critical.

***Love Is Never Jealous***

It is not possessive. True love allows the one you are dating to have freedom to express friendship with others of the opposite sex apart from your relationship. Jealousy is a sign of selfishness and insecurity.

***Love Is Never Boastful***

It is not on parade, always calling attention to itself. Love is "other" self-centered. When you really love someone, it's that person you brag about, not yourself.

***Love Is Not Proud***

Love gives you a humble spirit, not an arrogant, proud spirit. You are humbled that you are loved and humble in your loving.

***Love Is Never Haughty or Selfish***

Love thinks of others first. It is flexible enough to think of the plans of others. It can accept change in circumstances and people.

***Love Is Not Rude***

Love produces good manners and respect for others. Love in the heart produces good manners in words and actions.

### *Love Does Not Demand Its Own Way*

Love produces concern for the wants of the one being dated and the families involved.

### *Love Is Not Irritable or Touchy*

When we love someone we do not wear our feelings on our sleeve. We are not overly sensitive. We don't take everything personally.

### *Love Does Not Hold Grudges and Will Hardly Notice When Others Do It Wrong*

Love doesn't rehearse wrongs that have been done. Love forgets as well as forgives. It doesn't dwell on past failures.

### *Love Is Not Glad About Injustice*

Love takes no pleasure in the wickedness of other people. It is not joyously critical of faults.

### *Love Rejoices Whenever Truth Wins Out*

Love rejoices when good men do well. This is particularly true of dating. Love sees to it that truth is characteristic of the courtship.

### *Love Is Loyal No Matter What the Cost*

Love knows no limits to its patience. It believes in the person and his integrity. Love is loyal regardless.

### *You Will Always Believe in Him*

Love is not fickle. It trusts God to provide for the things lacking in the relationship.

***Always Expects the Best of Him***

Love always plays the "glad game." Love is very positive. It looks for the best and finds it.

***Always Stands Its Ground in Defending Him***

Love will continue to love even when that love is not returned. It does not seek reward, it only seeks to bless.

***On a Scale of One to Ten***

Now that you have examined the "real thing," how does your "love life" compare? Not too good, huh? Well, don't be too discouraged. You've just found a perfect "TEN." That's right, these verses describe God's perfect love. We don't love like that. We should, but we can't without His love in us to empower us. Yet, if you really love someone, the evidences of this love should be in your courtship. On a scale of one to ten, you should at least show up on the scale! No, zeros don't count! Real love can grow and mature toward perfection if it is present. However, if all you have is infatuation, it just can't produce deeds and attitudes of love. So, as you can see, there is a vast difference between love and infatuation.

# 34 Can a Teenager Really Be in Love?

As I mentioned earlier, one of my favorite questions in a dating seminar for young people is to ask them at what age they think a teenager is old enough to begin dating. The remarkable result is that the younger teenagers always feel that their age is the right age! All thirteen-year-olds vote for thirteen as minimum age. All the fourteen-year-olds believe they qualify. That's typical—and also very revealing. Older, and I might add, wiser, teenagers have the benefit of hindsight. They usually reserve dating for at least age sixteen or older. Why this caution by older teens? It seems by now they have learned from experience that dating demands some qualities often lacking during early adolescent years. Perhaps the one quality most needed in dating is the ability to love—genuinely—another person. Not every teenager (or adult, for that matter), is ready and able to love others. When are you capable of real love? Can a teenager be "in love"? Yes, he (or she) can, if that teenager can truly love himself. That's right: the ability to love others is determined by your own self-love.

### *Loving Your Neighbor*

One of God's great principles in the Bible is the second law: *Love your neighbor as you love yourself.* Have you ever really thought about that principle? I am commanded to love you (my neighbor) the same way I love myself. If I don't love myself, I can't love you. John Powell, in his wonderful little book *The Secret of Staying in Love* (Argus) says about this self-love: "I am sure that almost all human neuroses and moral evils stem from this one common cause: the absence of true love of one's self." That's a heavy statement but very true. Do you love yourself? Are you happy about yourself? Only when you are truly secure and happy about yourself are you able to love someone else.

***Self-love, Not Selfish Love***

The question then arises, What does it mean to love one's self? Isn't that selfish or self-centered? Not at all. The best way to answer that question is to ask another question. What does it mean to love another? Because loving yourself is like loving another. Loving another person means many things (as we discovered studying 1 Corinthians 13 in the preceding chapter), but, essentially, loving another means at least three things. Again I quote John Powell, who states in *The Secret of Staying in Love:*

1. Love esteems and affirms the unconditional and unique value of the one loved.
2. Love acknowledges and tries to fulfill the needs of the one loved.
3. Love forgives and forgets the failings of the one loved.

There is the essence of it. Loving my neighbor means that whatever I would do for you as my neighbor, I would also *do first* for myself. As Powell says, "It's a package deal. You have two people you must love—yourself and your neighbor." Take these three attitudes and apply them to yourself. Do you feel about yourself like that?

If you aren't able to give yourself this very special treatment, then you aren't able to give it to others. For example, do you really esteem your own unique value as a person? Are you able to accept yourself unconditionally? Second, do you understand that you yourself have legitimate needs and seek to meet them?

Are you able to forgive yourself for faults and failings? All these questions reveal your capacity to give love to others. Love your neighbor as you love yourself. Great advice.

### *Three Faces of Love*

We've spent some time defining love in the previous chapter, but another word might be enlightening. Teenagers are surrounded by our Cupid culture and the words *I love you* are common in youth dating experiences. In answer to this question about teenagers and love, it needs to be stressed that much of what we call love isn't the "forever" kind we talked about.

### *Greek Lovers*

The ancient Greeks must have been great lovers because they talked about love a great deal. In fact, they even had three words for love. These words were used to be very specific about the kind of love one was talking about. A look at these words can help us understand how we've abused our concept of love. The Greeks used the word *eros* to describe a passionate kind of love. *Eros* love is very common today and there is nothing wrong with passion; it just isn't deep enough for lasting commitment.

### *Possessive Love*

*Eros* is what we might call "I love you because of" kind of love. *Eros* says, "I love what you *have* and I want to possess it. I love your body, your car, your money, your fame. . . ." This passionate, possessive love isn't really love. It's centered on *me,* not you. It means I *want* you, not love you.

### *Conditional Love*

The Greeks had another word *philēo*, which was their word for friendly affection. Simon Peter used this word when talking to

Jews in John, chapter 21. Peter "loved" Jesus with a warm, friendly affection. That's good, but not good enough. Too many times *philēo* is a conditional love. The one receiving this love has to meet certain conditions. He has to perform, to qualify to receive it. It's an "I love you *if*" kind of love. I have to *do* something and do it right (by your standards) to get you to love me. This kind of love can do much hurt and harm. Erich Fromm, in his book *The Art of Loving* (Harper), says, ". . . to be loved because of one's merit, because one deserves it, always leaves doubt; maybe I did not please the person whom I want to love me, maybe this or that—there is always a fear that love could disappear. Furthermore, 'deserved' love easily leaves a bitter feeling that one is not loved for one's self, that one is loved *only* because one pleases. That one is, in the last analysis, not loved at all but used." Every child raised in a household where he had to "pay admission" to be accepted will grow up feeling unloved and insecure. Such a child has not been loved for himself and will in later years have trouble loving others unconditionally.

### *A Heavenly Word*

The Greeks had a third word which we've already looked at. This is the New Testament word *agape.* This is the unconditional love God has for us sinners. It is the "in spite of" love described in First Corinthians 13. This love is mature, selfless giving. Few teenagers, especially young teens, have this kind of love in their hearts. First of all, only God loves like that and His love must fill your heart continually to allow you to love this way.

This *in spite of* love is not unconditional. It does not need a worthy object. It just loves regardless. This is the love for which we all should strive. It is a blessing to receive it and an even greater blessing to be able to give it to others.

Finally, when is a teenager ready for love? A better question would be, when is *any person* ready to give love? In the words of a modern-day psychiatrist, Dr. Harry Stack Sullivan, in *Conceptions of Modern Psychiatry,* "When the satisfaction, security and development of another person becomes as significant to you as your own satisfaction, security, and development, love exists."

*There is your answer.*

*Love is a verb*
*Not just a noun.*
*Love is not a feeling*
*It is an action.*
*Love is something*
*You DO.*

# 35 How Do You Stay in Love After the Fireworks No Longer Go Off?

**I'VE SEEN SO MANY OF MY FRIENDS FALL IN AND OUT OF LOVE THAT I QUESTION THEIR JUDGMENT. I'VE NEVER BEEN IN LOVE, BUT WHEN LOVE COMES MY WAY, I WANT IT TO LAST. HOW DO YOU STAY IN LOVE AFTER THE FIREWORKS NO LONGER GO OFF?**

Starting power and staying power are seldom the same. It's not the runner who starts the race the fastest who always wins. It's the runner who finishes the fastest who gets the trophy. Being in love is like that. Honeymoons are great, wonderful, and a joy. However, when the honeymoon is over is when the work begins. Love is not something you "fall into" like a well. Love is not just a giggly feeling. Love is something you *do*. Love is more an act of the will than a feeling of the heart. Perhaps to further help us understand the secret of staying in love, we could offer some ideas about "forever" love that will be useful.

### *Love Is More Than a Feeling*

Feelings are fickle and change with circumstances. We feel blue on a rainy day; we feel good on a sunshiny day. Love is not like that. Love affects our feelings but is not bound by them. Love goes beyond the feeling to the living, in good times or bad.

### *Love Is Something You Do*

Erich Fromm writes, "Love is an activity, not a passive affect, it is a 'standing in,' not a 'falling for.' In the most general way, the active character of love can be described by stating that love is primarily *giving,* not receiving." Because love gives, it requires work and can be exhausting. To "love" many people would require great effort, perhaps too much. Therefore, you must choose whom you will love, and choose you can do. Love is a "will choice." How is this done? How do I choose? Generally, we choose those who share common interests and goals, or those who fulfill our needs. We even choose on the basis of those who give us good vibes. Choosing to love people who share our interests is always easier than loving those who differ with us. Loving the unlovely may require God's grace. Only God can love everyone. Remember, love can exist on many levels, therefore be careful not to offer a commitment of love beyond your intentions or capacity. We often do this under the influence of a full moon, a passionate embrace, or some other stimulant. John Powell says, "Immature people say things under the impulse of strong emotions which have a hollow sound the next morning after coffee" (from *The Secret of Staying in Love*).

### *Staying Love Is Unconditional*

Here is the fly in the ointment. Here is where most of us great "lovers" have our problem. Who can love unconditionally? I can't—not always. All of us, because we have been injured, scarred, or otherwise wounded, have our limitations. Only a totally unscarred and free person could continually give unconditional love. Such a person does not exist. Well, such a *human* person does not exist. Only *Jesus* can love like that. Therefore, this perfect *agape* love is a goal for which we strive, yes, even pray to receive as a gift from Him who is love itself. Without this unconditional love manifesting itself in dating, courtship, and marriage, the relationship cannot grow and deepen. The only kind of love that helps us grow and change is unconditional.

### *Staying Love Is Forever*

I've also heard it said that love works—*if* we will work at it. When we love unconditionally, we don't put time limits on our commitment. We don't say, "I'll love you until such and such." Love is permanent. It's pledged to last—forever. Such a pledge from you frees me to let go, reach out, and trust you.

Of course, to love someone forever is difficult or impossible, if that person doesn't respond to love. I have known people who gave love unconditionally for years with little or no response from the one loved. Such love can be hurt, bruised, and wounded. Should the one loved eventually respond and return the love, often the relationship is beyond repair.

### *Staying Love Builds Character*

Real love blesses those it touches. As I love you, my love empowers you to be yourself. It affirms and supports you. The proof of my love for you is not your esteem or admiration of me, but your appreciation of me for contributing to your own growth and personal worth. Love is in the *con*struction business, not the *de*struction business. My love for you helps you to love yourself and therefore to love others.

### *Staying Love Is an Open Hand*

Real love is not a closed fist, holding on. It is an open hand letting go. Love creates freedom; it is not possessive. In a courtship and marriage, unconditional love draws a couple closer and closer together, but as this closeness grows, it is not possessive. The trust and freedom create affirmation. A wise man once said,

"You did not come into this world to live up to my expectations. And I did not come into the world to live up to yours. If we meet, it will be beautiful. If we don't, it can't be helped." Too often in a courtship or marriage, we try to make the other into our own image, and love is crushed like a budding flower.

These, then, are some marks of a growing love relationship. There are many others, but these are needed and sufficient to show why some people who fall in love often fall out just as easily. It has been observed that the *second hardest* thing in all the world is to determine to involve one's self in the task of living intimately and growing with another. They say the *hardest* thing in all the world is to live alone. I believe this is true. Staying love is a risk, but it's worth the reach.

# 36 What About Being in Love With a Non-Christian?

**I'VE BEEN DATING A GUY WHO IS NOT A CHRISTIAN. I AM A VERY RELIGIOUS PERSON, AND SO IS MY FAMILY. MY PROBLEM IS, I THINK I'M IN LOVE WITH THIS GUY AND HE WANTS TO MARRY ME. CAN A CHRISTIAN BE IN LOVE WITH A LOST PERSON? WHAT DO YOU THINK?**

I think you need to think about some things that are very disturbing to me and later will be disturbing to you. Of course a Christian girl can love an unsaved guy. In fact, she should love everyone—but not the way you mean. When I hear the kind of question you're asking, I automatically want to ask some questions of my own. What kind of love are you talking about? What kind of Christian are you? What is it that you love about him? What kind of relationship do you have?

### *Christian—To What Degree?*

A Christian in love with a non-Christian has some problems, I think. Why? Because a Christian should have the mind of Christ. A Christian should show our Lord's values, goals, and purposes in life. A Christian woman "in love" with a lost guy ought to ask herself, "What am I in love with? Do I love him for his moral values, his determination to obey God, to seek first the Kingdom, and to be my spiritual leader?" Of course not. She loves none of these things about him, because they don't exist in a lost person's life. "A natural man does not accept the things of the Spirit of God; for they are foolishness to him . . ." (1 Corinthians 2:14). A "natural" man is the lost person—the unsaved, apart from God's grace. How can a person who loves God want to join her life to a man like that? What you love about him may be many worthy things such as his manliness, courage, tenderness, thoughtfulness, and strength, but these virtues are not worthy of a total commitment that marriage requires. Real love involves a oneness between two people in spiritual values and purposes.

***What Things in Common?***

It might be helpful if you evaluated your relationship in terms of your "fellowship." *Fellowship* is a great word because it means "things shared in common." What does a Believer share in common with a lost person? There are many areas of common interest that exist. Hobbies, music, sports, politics, intellectual interests, are all elements that could comprise fellowship between Christians and non-Christians. However, can you think of one single eternal value or interest they have in common? No, you can't. On the truly important areas such as God's will, God's ethics, God's Kingdom, God's family values, and God's husband-wife relationships, you find you two are near-strangers. Yet, it's in these areas that love and marriage exist. This is where real communication takes place. Paul asked a pertinent question in 2 Corinthians 6:14: ". . . what fellowship has light with darkness?"

***In Love With Love***

I guess what I'm saying is that, yes, you probably do love him—but not enough. You love him for the wrong reasons, which will not carry you through the troubled waters of your voyage together. Perhaps you are in love with love or the idea of being in love. At any rate, it's your decision to make. One good challenge from the psalmist may help: ". . . I desire no one on earth as much as you!" (Psalms 73:25 TLB). If you'll put God first, you'll *know* whether your love is right or wrong. I'll tell you something else: If you'll seek to desire no one on earth as much as Jesus, you begin to compare every man to Jesus. His personality will begin to shape your opinion of manhood. You'll begin to want your boyfriends to be like Christ. As you fall in love with your Lord, you'll find it more and more difficult to be "in love" with a man not like Him.

*Reputation is what people think you are.*
*Character is what you really are.*

*Coach John Wooden*

# 37 I'm Not Very Pretty and No Boys Will Date Me. What Can I Do?

**YOU ARE ALWAYS TALKING ABOUT DATING. I AM EIGHTEEN YEARS OLD AND I'VE NEVER HAD A DATE. NO BOY HAS EVER ASKED ME, AND I DON'T THINK ANYONE EVER WILL. I'M NOT VERY PRETTY. IN FACT, I'M FAT AND UGLY. I DON'T EVEN LIKE MYSELF. WHY WOULD ANY BOY WANT TO DATE ME?**

The above statement was turned in to me at a dating seminar recently. I've seen others like it before. My heart really goes out to a teenager like this. Often such statements come from boys as well as girls. "I'm ugly"—"I'm fat"—"Nobody likes me." These are the common expressions. How very sad that is. Everyone needs to feel loved, liked, and accepted. We cannot enjoy life without daily affirmation. John Powell says that people without a sense of self-appreciation can only suffer, and when one hurts with this pain, he hurts twenty-four uninterrupted hours a day. It is so important that each of us feels good about his or herself. A sense of worth is perhaps the most important attitude in life.

I once heard Bill Gothard ask us a penetrating question in a seminar on youth conflicts. Bill said, "If you could look in the magic mirror and change anything about your appearance, would you do so?" Most of us would recommend a complete overhaul! What would you change, your nose, weight, hair, height, or color? After asking us that question, Bill told us that if we would change anything in our basic appearance, that we were saying God made a mistake! What he meant was that when God made you and me, He had a plan and purpose for everything about us, even your too-large nose! To reject that idea is to reject your own self-hood. It is to live in discontent all your days.

### *Change What You Need to Change*

This does not mean that God is to be blamed for your being overweight. Your mouth did that! There are some aspects we can improve about our appearance that we ought to change for our own good and sense of well-being. Change what you can change, but accept yourself as God made you. If you are short—then believe God made you short for a purpose. Don't try to be tall by wearing elevator shoes and high cowboy hats! I like Evie's song: "I'm four-foot-eleven and going to heaven, and that makes me feel ten-feet tall!" All *right*—that's the attitude. What I'm saying is that before others can like and accept you, you must like and accept yourself. To do that, you must believe that Jesus loves you (made you) just as you are. To say you are ugly is one thing; to *feel* ugly is different. I may be ugly because I don't take care of my appearance. My clothes, hair, skin, and weight may all give evidence of my neglect. I may indeed look a mess. I may repel even my brother! However, usually people get in that kind of a mess because of the deeper problem—self-hatred.

### *Outside and Inside*

Usually the outside people see is merely the reflection of what we feel about ourselves on the inside. A happy heart makes for a glad countenance! A sad, dejected heart makes for a sad and sometimes fat, ugly, sloppy, or even depressed countenance. What is needed is a new feeling about yourself. You need to feel lovely and lovable so that others will see you that way also. Because if you don't develop this sense of self-worth, you are in real trouble.

Dr. William Glasser, author of *Reality Therapy,* makes some very keen remarks about a poor self-image. He says two crucial results come out of a lack of self-worth. First, Glasser says that *all* psychological problems have their roots in our need of a sense of personal worth. Second, he declares that the self-image you have of yourself will determine *all* of your behavior! People act (and especially relate) to other people, according to the way they think or feel about themselves.

Dr. Glasser goes on to affirm that when a good self-image is lacking, the results are very predictable. People who aren't happy about themselves seek destructions in order to survive. Work, television, play, all become substitutes for crying out, "Somebody love me!" They are attempted escapes from the pain of failure as a person. To the extent that you and I fail to perceive worth in ourselves, we will retreat into one of these "painkiller" solutions.

### *Tragic Results*

Often, if our hurt or rejection is great enough, even more tragic results occur. Depression, anger, and antisocial behavior, insanity, and even physical sickness are frequently the outward sign of inner hurt. It is commonly believed that 90 to 95 percent of all physical illness is psychologically caused. The fat person hates himself because he's fat, so he eats because he hates himself. It's a vicious circle. I'm hungry because I'm frustrated, and I'm frustrated because I eat too much!

### *Causes and Cures*

What I'm hoping we see is that in order to be loved, we must love ourselves. Once we feel good about ourselves, we are able to reach out to others. How does one find this sense of worth? How do broken-up people get put back together again? At the risk of sounding too simplistic, let me suggest a cure for the "uglies":

1. Realize God made you the way He wanted you.
2. Realize God's creation of you was and is perfect.
3. Realize God's love for you is constant and perfect.
4. Accept yourself because God accepts you.
5. Realize that beauty is in the eye of the beholder. You are as attractive as you feel you are. God thinks you are the greatest. Agree with Him and act accordingly.
6. Start giving love to others. Love flows outward. Give it in order to get it. He who would have friends must first be a friend to others.

# 38 How Can I Get Someone I Really Like to Like Me?

Does "like me" mean "love me"? When teenagers talk about she *likes* me, I think I know what they are saying but I'm not sure. I'm not sure *they* know. It seems we're talking about infatuation, not love. "Liking" a girl or boy romantically has to do with physical attraction, which makes our glands work but doesn't do much for human relationships.

What I suggest is that you forget about getting someone to "like" you, and begin to work on getting to know the wonderful person. If a girl is "crazy" about a boy, and he doesn't even know she exists, what can she do?

## *God Isn't Cupid*

If she is a Christian (and a lady), there are some actions she shouldn't take, as we've already stated earlier in this book; flirting is a no-no. She doesn't have to phone him or pass him notes in class with perfume sprinkled on them (that's too expensive). She doesn't need to "parade" her assets before his eyes either. Also, praying to God to make him notice her probably won't influence heaven's angels to zap the poor guy with an arrow dipped in love potion. God doesn't play Cupid for anybody, not even you. However, He does care about your friendships and whom you love.

***To Have a Friend***

What I suggest is that you become a friend to your dreamboat. Get to know him (her) by going to the same places, doing group things together. The only way to get a friend is to become one. As the two of you grow in friendship, the "liking" thing either will happen or it will not. If it doesn't, sigh really deep, expel your love, and move on to other prospects. Nothing ventured, nothing gained. Right?

# 39 Is Premarital Sex Wrong for Engaged Couples If It's an Expression of Real Love?

**I AM ENGAGED AND MY FIANCÉE AND I PLAN TO BE MARRIED IN A FEW MONTHS. WE'VE BEEN HAVING SEX FOR SOME TIME NOW. WE FEEL MARRIED, ALL WE LACK IS THAT PIECE OF PAPER. I DON'T FEEL OUR SEX IS WRONG, BECAUSE IT COMES OUT OF OUR LOVE. WHAT DO YOU THINK?**

I think you are mistaken. I think you are sincere—but sincerely wrong. I also think your experience is fairly common, even among Christian young adults. Because we cannot always trust what we feel to lead us to the truth; I need to add some thoughts here that might help you.

Obviously some couples, when truly in love, feel little or no guilt about premarital sex. This "feeling married" is sufficient for the time being, until the "legal papers" are secured.

### *Degrees of Promiscuity*

To begin with, I agree with Tim Stafford, quoted earlier, that God doesn't classify sex between engaged couples as He does casual sex with a near-stranger. Sin is sin, but there is a difference between a bum stealing a ride on a railroad, and another bum of a different type stealing the whole railroad! Both are stealing, but one to a greater degree. However, why should there be any question about premarital sex being right or wrong? God's Word has stated clearly, "flee fornication." "Fornication and indecency of any kind . . . must not be so much as mentioned among you, as befits the people of God" (Ephesians 5:3 NEB). Does being in love or engaged somehow right the immoral sex act? Promiscuity is not baptized and made holy by the love motive. Be very careful here. Love does not make all things right—obedience is a factor. We can be fooled by our emotions. Better to obey God's Word. Again, a good word here comes from John White's *Eros Defiled:*

> But love that fulfills the law is not the glazed, heavy-breathed stirring in the groins that clouds your judgment and seduces your will as you copulate. It is not love that you *make.* Premarital sexual excitement too often becomes all-important, as many unmarried people have discovered. It blocks the very communication it is designed to promote.

This is wisdom. Just because you and your lover have made promises to each other does not mean that those promises are the same as or equal to marriage. Marriage vows and contracts are public and legal promises of commitment. When an engaged couple (or even a couple who have promised love with no mention publicly of marriage) have sex, this is not the same as being married. Don't be misled here. Private promises of the heart are not the same as public promises made before God and man at a wedding altar. Marriage is much more than a "piece of paper."

### *But It Feels So Right*

I can just hear you now, "But it feels so right. . . ." I'm sure it does. Your conscience has been defiled. You've rationalized away the sin of it. You've made your own ethic here. Again, I'm not saying your sex is not an act of love. I'm not saying it isn't meaningful or wholesome. I'm not trying to make it dirty. However, feeling right about something doesn't make it right, now does it? A feeling of rightness proves nothing except to the person who wants it to. You may be doing a good thing in a bad way (sex without marriage). You've settled for less than the best, and you may be very sorry later on. There just isn't a right way to do a wrong thing.

# Glossary

*ABORTION*

In layman's terms, an abortion is an external interruption of a live pregnancy inside the female uterus, causing the pregnancy to pass to the outside. Technically, there are two ways this can be accomplished: it can be either a medical abortion performed by qualified medical staff; or it can be a nonmedical abortion performed by a nonqualified person (or persons). All abortions entail some risk to the mother. The degree of risk is determined by how long the pregnancy is allowed to continue and by whom the abortion is administered. (See *Abortion: The Personal Dilemma,* R. F. Gardner, Spire Books, 1974.)

*ADULTERY*

Sexual intercourse outside the marriage vows with another man's wife or husband, or sex between a married person and a single person.

*CHASTITY BELT*

Webster's defines as "a securely fastened, beltlike device of metal, leather, or other material, worn by women in the Middle Ages to prevent sexual intercourse during the absence of their husbands."

*CLEAR CONSCIENCE*

The ability to face another person without guilt for past or unforgiven offenses (Matthew 5:23,24).

*CONCUPISCENCE*

An old English word used in the King James Version (1 Thessalonians 4:5) which describes a person whose sensual passions far outweigh their spiritual desires.

*DATING*

A special kind of friendship between two people of the opposite sex that may lead to courtship, love, and marriage.

*DEFRAUDING*

Another King James Version word describes sexual activity outside God's moral plan. Bill Gothard defines defrauding as "arousing sensual desires in others which cannot be righteously satisfied."

*FONDLE*

Generally known as "touching" the sex organs as a part of petting or foreplay. The Bible calls such activity among the nonmarried "defrauding" (2 Thessalonians 4:6).

*FORNICATION*

From the biblical word *porneia* in Greek. Our English word *porno* or *pornographic* comes from this word. It means sexual intercourse outside of marriage. Strictly speaking, it is to be distinguished from adultery, yet it can include adultery. Fornication is sex between unmarried people. It is translated in the New American Standard Bible by the broader idea of sexual immorality of any kind (1 Thessalonians 4:3).

*JEALOUSY*

A deliberate desire to deprive others of pleasures that might draw them away from you (Proverbs 6:34).

*LASCIVIOUSNESS*

King James Version. An old word describing a depraved life and heart. It describes a person whose whole life is sensual and sexual. Someone called it the "ugliest" word in the Bible.

*LUST*

An "overdesire." Sexual lust would be any sexual thought or action motivated by selfishness, which is potentially destructive to others and which dishonors God. Lust is taking; love is giving.

*MASTURBATION*

Physically stimulating yourself sexually by manipulating your sexual organs, usually to the point of orgasm (sex release). Although not considered by some a sin in and of itself, self-manipulation, when habitual and accompanied by fantasies of exotic mental images, can be damaging emotionally as well as sinful. As one author put it, "No other form of sexual activity has been so frequently discussed, so soundly condemned, and more universally practiced, than masturbation." (Quote from L. Dearborn's "Autoeroticism" in *The Encyclopedia of Sexual Behavior* [Eds. A. Ellis and Aborbane] Vol. 1, 204, Hawthorn Books, NY.)

*ORAL SEX*

Sexual gratification, using the lips and tongue of the man or woman to caress the genital organs.

*PEER PRESSURE*

A sociologist's term describing the effect of environment on behavior. Your peers are those in your own social life who influence your behavior collectively. A group culture puts "pressure" on the individual to conform to the group's behavior and culture.

*PROMISCUOUS*

From the Latin *Miscere* meaning "mixed." Thus, mixed or unrestrained sexual activity—sexual desires run wild without regard to God's standards.

*SENSUALITY*

Planned appeal to the physical senses for personal gratification.

*TEMPTATIONS*

Situations designed by Satan to lead us into sin.